THE LARYNGECTOMEE GUIDE

EXPANDED EDITION

Itzhak Brook, M.D., M.Sc.

ISBN: 9781976852398

TABLE OF CONTENTS

Dedication

The guide is dedicated to my fellow laryngectomees and their caregivers for their courage and perseverance.

Acknowledgement

I am most grateful to Joyce Reback Brook for her editorial assistance.

Disclaimer

Dr. Brook is not an expert in otolaryngology and head and neck surgery. This guide is not a substitute for medical care by medical professionals.

INTRODUCTION

I am a physician who became a laryngectomee in 2008. I was diagnosed with laryngeal cancer in 2006 and was initially treated with a course of radiation. After experiencing a recurrence two years later, my doctors recommended that total laryngectomy was the best assurance for eradicating the cancer. As I write this, it has been ten years since my operation; there has been no sign of recurrence.

After becoming a laryngectomee, I realized the magnitude of the challenges faced by new laryngectomees in learning how to care for themselves. Overcoming these challenges requires mastering new techniques in caring for one's airways, dealing with life long side effects of radiation and other treatments, living with the results of surgeries, facing uncertainties about the future, and struggling with psychological, social, medical and dental issues. I also learned the difficulties of life as a head and neck cancer survivor. This cancer and its treatment affect some of the most basic human functions, communication, nutrition, and social interaction.

As I gradually learned to cope with my life as a laryngectomee, I realized that the solutions to many problems are not only based on medicine and science but also on experience in addition to trial and error. I also realized that what works for one person may not always work for another. Because each person's medical history, anatomy and personality are different, so are some of the solutions. However, some general principles of care are helpful to most laryngectomees. I was fortunate to benefit from my physicians, speech and language pathologists, and other laryngetomees as I learned how to care for myself and overcome the myriad of daily challenges.

I gradually realized that new and even seasoned laryngectomees would probably improve their quality of life from learning how to better care for themselves. To that end I created a Website (http://dribrook.blogspot.com/) to help laryngectomees and other individuals with head and neck cancer. The site deals with medical, dental and psychological issues and also contains links to videos about rescue breathing and other informative lectures.

This practical guide is based on my Website and is aimed at providing practical information that can assist laryngectomees and their caregivers in dealing with medical, dental and psychological issues. The guide contains information about the side effects of radiation and chemotherapy; the methods of speaking after laryngectomy; how to care for the airways, stoma, heat and moisture exchange filter, and voice prosthesis. In addition I address eating and swallowing issues, medical, dental and psychological concerns, respiration and anesthesia, and travelling as a laryngectomee.

The expanded edition of the guide is an updated and expanded version of the earlier 2013 edition. It contains additional information on most topics, describes newer devices and products that are available for laryngectomee care.

This guide is not a substitute for professional medical care but hopefully will be useful for laryngectomees and their caregiver(s) in dealing with their lives and the challenges they face.

Chapter 1:

Risk factors, diagnosis and treatment of primary and recurrent laryngeal and other head and neck cancer cancers

Risk factors of head and neck cancers

- **Alcohol and tobacco use.** The two major risk factors for developing head and neck cancers (HNC) are alcohol and tobacco use. This is especially true for cancers of the oral cavity, oropharynx, hypopharynx, and larynx (not salivary gland cancers). It is estimated that at least 75% of head and neck cancers are caused by tobacco and alcohol use. Using both tobacco and alcohol places people at higher risk for developing these cancers.

- **Human papillomavirus (HPV)** is a risk factor for some HNC, especially oropharyngeal involving the tonsils or the base of the tongue.

- **Epstein-Barr virus infection.** Infection with the Epstein-Barr virus is a risk factor for nasopharyngeal and salivary glands cancers.

- **Radiation exposure.** Radiation to the head and neck, for noncancerous conditions or cancer, is a risk factor for salivary glands cancer.

- **Oral health.** Poor oral hygiene, missing teeth, and using mouthwash with a high alcohol content are risk factors for oral cavity cancer.

- **Preserved or salted foods.** Consumption of certain preserved or salted foods during childhood is a risk factor for nasopharyngeal cancer.

- **Paan (betel quid).** Sometimes used in Southeast Asia is strongly associated with an increased risk of oral cancer.

- **Occupational exposure.** Wood dust is a risk factor for nasopharyngeal cancer. Asbestos, synthetic fibers, metal, textile, ceramic, and logging have been associated with cancer of the larynx. Wood, nickel dust, and formaldehyde may increase risk for cancer of the paranasal sinuses and nasal cavity.

- **Ancestry.** Asian ancestry, particularly Chinese, is a risk factor for nasopharyngeal cancer.
- **Maté.** A tea-like beverage consumed by South Americans has been associated with an increased risk of cancers of the mouth, throat, esophagus, and larynx.

Overview

Laryngeal cancer affects the voice box. Cancers that start in the larynx are called laryngeal cancers; cancers of the hypopharynx are called **hypopharyngeal cancers**. The hypopharynx is the part of the throat (pharynx) that lies beside and behind the larynx. (**Figure 1**) These cancers are very close to each other and the treatment principles of both are similar and may involve laryngectomy. Although the discussion below addresses laryngeal cancer, it is also generally applicable to hypopharyngeal cancer.

Laryngeal cancer occurs when malignant cells appear in the larynx. The larynx contains the vocal folds (or cords) which, by vibrating generate sounds that create audible voice when the vibrations echo through the throat, mouth, and nose.

The larynx is divided into three anatomical regions: the glottis (in the middle of the larynx, includes the vocal cords); the supraglottis (in the top part and includes the epiglottis, arytenoids and aryepiglottic folds, and false cords); and the subglottis (in the bottom of the larynx). While cancer can develop in any part of the larynx, most laryngeal cancers originate in the glottis. Supraglottic cancers are less common, and subglottic tumors are the least frequent.

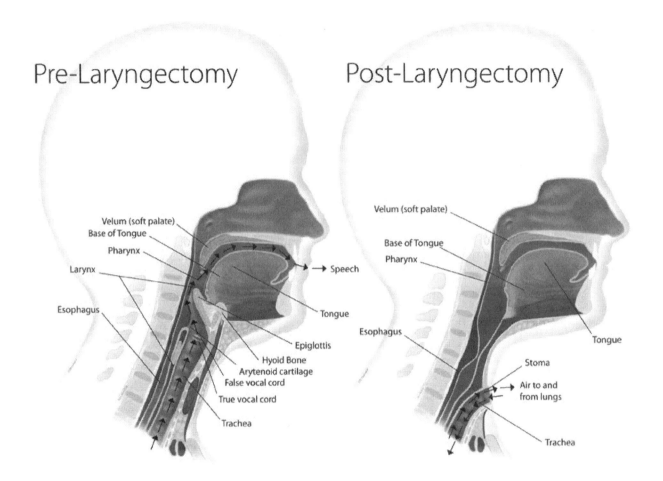

Figure 1: Anatomy of the larynx before and after laryngectomy

Laryngeal and hypopharyngeal cancer may spread by direct extension to adjacent structures, by metastasis to regional cervical lymph nodes, or more distantly, through the blood stream to other locations in the body. Distant metastases to the lungs and liver are most common. Squamous cell carcinomas account for 90 to 95 percent of laryngeal and hypopharyngeal cancer.

Smoking, and heavy alcohol consumption are the main risk factors for laryngeal cancer. Exposure to human papilloma virus (HPV) has been mainly associated with oropharyngeal cancer and to a lesser degree with laryngeal and hypopharyngeal ones.

There are about 50,000 to 60,000 laryngectomees in the USA. According to the Surveillance Epidemiology and End Results Cancer Statistics Review of the National Cancer Institute, an estimated 12,250 men and women are diagnosed with cancer of the larynx each year. The number of new laryngectomees has been declining mainly because fewer people are smoking and newer therapeutic approaches can spare the larynx.

Diagnosis

Symptoms and signs of laryngeal cancer include:

- Abnormal (high-pitched) breathing sounds
- Chronic cough (with and without blood)
- Difficulty swallowing
- A sensation of a lump in the throat
- Hoarseness that does not get better in 1-2 weeks
- Neck and ear pain
- Sore throat that does not get better in 1-2 weeks, even with antibiotics
- Swelling or lumps in the neck that does not heal
- Unintentional weight loss

The symptoms associated with laryngeal cancer depend upon its location. Persistent hoarseness can be the initial complaint in cancers of the glottis. Later symptoms may include difficulty in swallowing, ear pain, chronic and sometimes bloody cough, and hoarseness. Supraglottic cancers are frequently diagnosed only when they cause airway obstruction or palpable metastatic lymph nodes. Primary subglottic tumors typically present with hoarseness or complaints of difficulty in breathing on exertion.

There is no single test that can accurately diagnose cancer. The complete evaluation of a patient generally requires a thorough history and physical examination along with diagnostic testing. Many tests are required to determine if a person has cancer or if another condition (such as an infection) may be mimicking the symptoms of cancer.

Effective diagnostic testing is used to confirm or eliminate the presence of cancer, monitor its progress, and plan for and evaluate the effectiveness of treatment. In some instances, it is necessary to perform repeat testing if a person's condition has changed, a sample collected was not of good quality, or an abnormal test result needs to be confirmed. Diagnostic procedures for cancer may include imaging, laboratory tests, tumor biopsy, endoscopic examination, surgery, or genetic testing.

The following tests and procedures may be used to help diagnose and stage laryngeal cancer which influences the choice of treatment:

- **Physical examination** of the throat and neck: This enables the doctor to feel for swollen lymph nodes in the neck and to view the throat by using a small, long-handled mirror to check for abnormalities.
- **Endoscopy:** A procedure by which an endoscope (a flexible lighted tube) is inserted through the nose or mouth into the upper airway to the larynx, enabling the examiner to directly view these structures.
- **Laryngoscopy:** A procedure to examine the larynx with a mirror or a laryngoscope (a rigid lighted tube).
- **CT scan (computed tomography):** A procedure that generates a series of detailed radiographs of body sites, taken from different directions. A contrast material such as an injected or swallowed dye enables better visualization of the organs or tissues.
- **MRI (magnetic resonance imaging)**: A procedure that uses a magnet and radio waves to generate a series of detailed pictures of areas inside the body.
- **Barium swallow:** A procedure to examine the esophagus and stomach. The patient drinks a barium solution that coats the esophagus and stomach, and X-rays are obtained.
- **Biopsy:** A procedure where tissues are obtained so that they can be viewed under a microscope to check for cancer.

The potential for recovery from laryngeal cancer depends on the following:

- The extent the cancer has spread (the "stage")
- The appearance of the cancer cells (the "grade")

- The location(s) and size of the tumor
- The patient's age, gender, and general health

Additionally, smoking tobacco and drinking alcohol decrease the effectiveness of treatment for laryngeal cancer. Patients with laryngeal cancer who continue to smoke and drink are less likely to be cured and more likely to develop a second tumor.

Treatment of throat and laryngeal cancers

Individuals with early or small throat or laryngeal cancer may be treated with surgery or radiation therapy (RT). Those with advanced or recurrent cancer may require a combination of treatments. This may include surgery as well as a combination of RT and chemotherapy generally given at the same time.

Some patients may benefit from second-line therapies that include immunotherapy using checkpoint inhibitors, and anti-epidermal growth factor receptor (EGFR) monoclonal antibodies.

Checkpoint inhibitors block normal proteins on cancer cells, or the proteins on the T cells that respond to them. These agents strive to overcome one of cancer's main defenses against the individual's immune system attack.

Targeted therapy is another therapeutic option specifically directed at advanced laryngeal cancer. Targeted cancer therapies are administered by using drugs or other substances that block the growth and spread of cancer by interfering with specific molecules involved in tumor growth and progression.

The treatment recommendations that are given for a particular individual's treatment are usually decided at a Tumor Board team conference where a decision is made usually in accordance with evidence-based guidelines from the National Comprehensive Cancer Network (NCCN).Selection of the treatment regimen takes into consideration the location of the tumor, and whether the cancer has spread to other sites, previous treatment history, patient's general state and other medical problems, and the potential regimen's toxicities.

A team of medical specialists generally collaborate in planning the treatment. These can include:

- Ear, nose, and throat doctor(s) (otolaryngologists)
- General head and neck surgeon(s)
- Medical oncologist(s)
- Radiation oncologist(s)

Other health care providers who work with the specialists as a team may include a dentist, plastic surgeon, reconstructive surgeon, speech and language pathologist, oncology nurse, dietitian, and a mental health counselor. It is best to have a patient care coordinator that develops, monitors, and evaluates the interdisciplinary care.

Treatment options depend on the following:

- The extent to which the cancer has spread (the stage)
- The location and size of the tumor
- Whether the cancer has return
- Maintaining the patient's ability to talk, eat, and breathe as normally as possible
- The patient's general health
- Potential side effects and toxicities

Other factors that may be considered include distance to the treatment center, need for follow-up care, and the availability of certain procedures at the local facility.

The medical team describes the available treatment choices to the patient and the expected results, as well as the possible side effects. Patients should carefully consider available options and understand how these treatments may affect their ability to eat, swallow, and talk, and whether the treatments will alter their appearance during and after treatment. The patient and his/her health care team can work together to develop a treatment plan that fits the patient's needs and expectations.

Supportive care for control of pain and other symptoms that can relieve potential side effects and ease emotional concerns should be available before, during, and after cancer treatment.

Patients should be well informed before making their choice. If necessary obtaining a second medical and/or surgical opinion is helpful. Patients are often stressed and anxious when they learn that they suffer from a serious illness and may not be able to integrate all the information and explanations they hear. They may therefore need to hear these several times to integrate the information. Having a patient advocate (family member or friend) attend the discussions with the medical team is desirable as they can assist the patient in making the best choice.

It is suggested to ask the following questions of the treatment team:

- What is the size, location, spread, and stage of the tumor?
- What is the HPV status of the cancer?
- What are the treatment options? Would they include surgery, radiation therapy, chemotherapy or a combination of these? Is laryngectomy the only viable option?
- What are the expected side effects, risks and benefits of each kind of treatment?
- How can side effects be managed?
- What is the risk of recurring cancer?
- What will be the sound of the voice following each of the above treatments?
- What are the chances of being able to eat normally?
- How will the breathing be affected?
- How to prepare for treatment?
- Will the treatment require hospitalization and if so for how long?
- What is the estimated cost of the treatment and will insurance cover it?
- How will the treatment affect one's life, work and normal activities?
- Is a research study (clinical trial) a good option?

- Can the physician recommend an expert for a second opinion regarding the treatment options?
- How often and for how long will there be a need for follow ups?
- Is there a support group in the area that can assist after surgery?

What to tell your physician

To help one's physicians provide the best care it is helpful to provide them with this information:

- Detailed past medical, dental, social and psychological history
- Detailed description about your symptoms
- Any handicap you have
- Past surgeries
- Past vaccinations
- Medications you take
- Your diet
- Illnesses in your family
- Your work, and travel history (not only recent)
- Exposure to irritants, toxins etc.
- Allergies to food and medications
- Your life style, daily activities, and long term plans
- List of all the physicians and medical care providers
- Your preferred treatment (after hearing the options)
- Your preference knowing details on your condition, treatment and prognosis
- Your preferences about life support
- Your medical insurance coverage

It is a useful to prepare a list of all these issues ahead of time and hand it over to one's physician and other medical providers.

Dealing with psychological and social issues

Learning that one has laryngeal or any head and neck cancer can change the individual's life and the lives of those close to them. These changes can be difficult to deal with. Getting help to better cope with the psychological and social impact of the diagnosis is very important.

The emotional burden includes concerns about treatment and its side effects, hospital stays, and the economic impact of the illness including how to deal with medical bills. Additional worries are directed at how to care for one's family, keep one's work, and continue one's daily activities.

Sources for support include members of the health care team who can answer and clarify questions about treatment, work, or other activities. Social workers, counselors, or members of the clergy can be helpful if one wishes to share his/her feelings or concerns. Social workers can suggest resources for financial aid, transportation, home care, and emotional support. Support groups may also offer support in person, over the telephone, or on the Internet. Member of the health care team can help in finding support groups.

Diagnosis and treatment of recurrent cancer

Recurrent cancer can occur near the original site of the tumor, known as recurrent local-regional cancer, or at distant sites in the body, known as recurrent metastatic cancer. Squamous cell carcinomas of the oropharynx associated with human papillomavirus (HPV) usually have better outcomes that those not associated with HPV. Patients with these cancers experience a later onset of distant metastasis and more metastatic sites in atypical locations. The symptoms of recurrent cancer can be similar to the primary one or different depending on its location.

Recurrent head and neck cancer is more challenging and difficult than the initial cancer. Treatment options, course and goals depend on whether the recurrence is local, regional or metastatic.

The treatment options used for local or regional recurrent head and neck cancer are similar to those used for newly diagnosed disease. These include: surgery, radiation therapy, chemoradiation therapy, chemotherapy, immunotherapy, and targeted agents. However, previously treatment with RT will influence current treatment choices as it may exclude the patient from additional radiation treatment. However, re-irradiation is possible in some selected cases. Re-irradiation is more challenging than initial treatment because of the side effects of prior therapy and concerns about the risks of high cumulative radiation doses to normal structures.

Unfortunately, the prognosis for recurrent metastatic head and neck cancer is not good. The goals of treatment for recurrent metastatic disease are either to reduce disease symptoms (palliative care), such as pain, and/or to improve survival. Sometime a clinical trial is an optional treatment course. These trials can allow access to new therapies not available to most health care providers or patients, even if it has not yet been determined if the novel therapies will improve outcomes including survival. Decisions about the treatment goals and optimal course of treatment should be made with the patient's participation.

Chapter 2:

Having surgery: types of laryngectomy and reconstruction, outcome, recovery, survival, pain management and seeking a second opinion.

Types of surgery including laryngectomy

Treatment of laryngeal cancer often includes surgery. The surgeon can use either scalpel or laser. Laser surgery is performed using a device that generates an intense beam of light that cuts or destroys tissues.

There are two types of surgery for removal of laryngeal cancer:

- **Removal of part of the larynx (partial laryngectomy):** The surgeon takes out only the part of the larynx harboring the tumor.
- **Removal of the entire larynx (total laryngectomy):** The surgeon removes the whole larynx and some adjacent tissues.

Total laryngectomy is generally performed for these reasons:

- A large laryngeal untreated cancer that has eroded through cartilage and other structures.
- Laryngeal cancer that came back after previous treatment, (i.e., radiation with/without chemotherapy).
- Prevention of aspiration pneumonia resulting from prior head and neck cancer surgery at sites other the larynx (i.e., hypopharynx, tongue base).
- Nonfunctional larynx, or inability to eat or drink because of pharyngeal or esophageal strictures.

Lymph nodes that are close or drain the cancerous site may also be taken out during either type of surgery.

The patient may need to undergo reconstructive or plastic surgery to rebuild the affected tissues. The surgeon may obtain tissues from other parts of the body to repair the site of the surgery in the throat and/or neck. The reconstructive or plastic surgery may take place at the same time when the cancer is removed, or it can be performed later on.

Healing after surgery, and the length of time needed to recover varies among individuals.

Surgical reconstruction in total laryngectomy

Total laryngectomy is an effective and reliable operation used to remove advanced cancer of the larynx, especially when conservative approaches were unsuccessful. The defect created after the larynx is removed is generally easy to close using sutures or staples. However, when the tumor has spread beyond the larynx and also involves the pharynx or esophagus, such closure is no longer possible and more complex reconstructive options have to be used.

The purpose of reconstruction is to recreate an effective passage through which swallowing as well as esophageal or tracheoesophageal speech are possible. Surgical reconstruction increases surgical time, cost, and postsurgical risks.

When additional tissue is needed to correct the defect, the reconstructive method is affected by the size of the defect, which determines the amount of tissue needed to repair it. The tissue used is called a "flap". Flaps can be regional (obtained from a site close to the defect) or distal (obtained from a site some distance away from the defect). The blood supply to the flap can either be kept intact (in the regional flap), or the artery and vein serving it need to be connected to the blood supply at the location where it is required. These types of flaps as called "free flaps".

The types of available flaps are:

Regional flaps

- Pectoralis myocutaneous (PMC) flap.
- Deltopectoral (DP) flap.

Free flaps

- Radial forearm free flap (RFFF)
- Jejunal free flap (JFF)

Pectoralis myocutaneous. This flap has been used for many years and originates from the muscle of the chest and the skin above it. Its advantages are: the excellent and reliable blood supply, availability of sufficient amount of tissue, and proximity to the neck. Its disadvantages include: its large size, the cosmetic deformity it creates by transposing it under the neck skin, and the weakness of the arm it may create.

Deltopectoral flap. Tissues for this flap are taken from deltopectoral muscles region. It is thinner and more closely fits the thin tissue of the pharynx. DP creates minimal donor site problems, but installation of the flap may need to be completed in several stages, and the amount of tissue that can be obtained maybe limited.

Radial forearm free flap. A larger more pliable flap is needed when parts the pharynx or esophagus are removed. This may require using a radial forearm which is obtained from the inside surface of the arm near the wrist. The artery and vein that serve the flap have to be sewn to an artery and vein in the neck (a microvascular anastomosis). The donor site is covered with a skin graft taken from another site. This procedure can compromise the blood supply to the hand in individuals with poor hand circulation, and this risk is evaluated prior to considering the RFFF. The first two weeks following surgery are the most vulnerable to blood supply interruption as the new blood supply may clot of. Such interruption has to be addressed promptly to prevent the flap from dying.

Taking one's pulse at the wrist is no longer possible after the surgery. It is important to notify one's medical providers about this.

The jejunal free flap. The JFF is an alternative to the RFFF. It comes as a cylinder and is especially useful when parts of the esophagus are removed. Although swallowing is generally adequate, the voice is less good as with the RFFF.

In instances where all of the pharynx, larynx, and esophagus are taken out, the stomach can be connected directly to the throat. Because of the potential for a serious infection in the mediastinum after this surgery it is generally used in the most advanced cases where no alternative for reconstruction is available.

The reconstructive options currently available allow for the treatment of more advanced cancer, with a higher likelihood of successful restoration of voicing and swallowing than has been possible in the past. The best option for the patient depends on the tumor's extent, the risks of each reconstructive option, and the patient's overall health. Discussion between the patients and surgeon of the risks and benefits of each option can assist in selecting the best one. Obtaining a second option can also assist in the process.

Preparing for surgery

Prior to surgery it is important to thoroughly discuss with the surgeon all available therapeutic and surgical options and their short and long term outcomes. Patients scheduled for surgery may be anxious and under a lot of stress. It is therefore important to have a patient advocate (such as a family member or friend) also attend the meetings with the surgeon. It is important to freely ask and discuss any concerns and request clarifications. It is necessary to repeatedly listen to explanations until they are understood. It is useful to prepare questions to ask the surgeon and write down the information obtained.

In addition to consultation with the surgeon, it is also important to see these medical providers:

- Internist and/or family physician
- Any specialist one sees for a specific medical problem (i.e. cardiologist, pulmonologis, etc.)
- Medical oncologist
- Radiation oncologist
- Anesthetist
- Dentist
- Speech and language pathologist (SLP)
- Social worker or mental health counselor
- Nutritionist

Pre-operative counseling sessions with the patient and family are essential in clarifying what to expect regarding communication restoration. It is also very useful to meet other patients who have already undergone a laryngectomy. These individuals can guide the patient about future speech options, share some of their experiences and provide emotional support.

The speech and language pathologist (SLP) plays an important role in the care of the total laryngectomy patients from initiation of pre-operative counseling through acute care, home health and outpatient services. These includes the pre-laryngectomy evaluation and education; immediate post-operative care, post-surgical home care; and post-operative outpatient care.

Contacting a local laryngectomee club to meet other laryngectomees and find support before and after the surgery can be helpful. Lists of local laryngectomee clubs, and SLP that take care of laryngectomees is available at the International Association of Laryngectomee website. (http://theial.com/)

Getting a second opinion

When facing a new medical diagnosis that requires making a choice between several therapeutic options including surgery, it is important to get a second opinion. There may be different medical and surgical approaches and a second (or even third) opinion may be invaluable. Getting such an opinion from physicians experienced in the issues at hand is judicious. There are many situations when treatment cannot be reversed. This is why choosing the course of therapy after consulting with at least one more specialist is very important.

Some individuals may be reluctant to ask for a referral to see another physician for a second opinion. Some may be afraid that this will be interpreted as lack of confidence in their primary physician or doubts about their competence. However, most clinicians welcome and encourage the practice and many medical insurers welcome it.

The second doctor may agree with the first doctor's diagnosis and treatment plan. Conversely, the other physician may suggest a different approach. Either way, the patient ends up with more valuable information and also with a greater sense of control. Eventually one may feel more confident about the decisions he/she makes, knowing that all options have been considered.

Gathering one's medical records and seeing another physician may take some time and effort. Generally, the delay in initiating treatment will not make the eventual treatment less effective. However, one should discuss any possible delay with the physician.

There are numerous ways to find an expert for a second opinion. One can request a referral to another specialist from the primary doctor, a local or state medical society, a nearby hospital, or a medical school. Even though patients with cancer are often in a rush to get treated and remove the cancer as soon as possible-waiting for another opinion may be worthwhile.

Recovery from surgery

The patient's course of recover depends on the extent of the surgery and reconstruction. After some surgeries, it is possible to be discharged after several hours of observation in the recovery room, while other surgeries may require a hospital stay for 7 to 14 days. A longer stay may be needed because of post-operative complications.

Hospital recovery takes place in different parts of the medical center. Patients are first observed in the recovery room, than they are moved to the intensive care unit, and lastly to the regular surgical or otolaryngological ward. Each move is made when the time is right. With time the lines, tubes, catheters and drains are gradually removed, and the patient is eventually helped to get up and walk.

The post-surgical risks following laryngectomy include: local bleeding (including hematoma), infection, salivary fistula, low calcium levels (hypocalcemia), hypothyroidism, blood clots, and aspiration (after partial laryngectomy).

Patients are discharge from the hospital once the physician(s) determine that there is no longer a need for in-patient level care. Some patients can go home directly from the hospital with or without visiting nurses; others might need to be transferred to a rehabilitation or skilled nursing facility before going home. Selection of the best discharge location is made by the medical team that is made of physicians, social workers, nurses and physical therapists. It is made in conjunction with the patient and his/her family.

A speech and language pathologist is also involved to assisting the patient to learn about speaking options. Patients should be informed about the need for continued speech rehabilitation and communication options post-operatively.

Further reconstructive and cosmetic procedures or treatments are generally done after discharge. This allows time for recovery from the initial surgery, get the pathological results from specimens obtained during the surgery, and make any arrangements needed for the next steps.

Surgery's outcome

The surgery can result in all or some of the following:

- Throat and neck swelling
- Local pain
- Tiredness
- Increased mucus production
- Changes in physical appearance
- Numbness, muscle stiffness and weakness
- Tracheostomy

Most people feel weak or tired for some time after surgery, have a swollen neck, and experience pain and discomfort for the first few days. Pain medications can relieve some of these symptoms.

Surgery can alter the ability to swallow, eat, or talk. However, not all such effects are permanent, as discussed in **Chapter 11**. Those who lose their ability to talk after surgery may find it useful to communicate by writing on a notepad, writing board (such as a magic slate), smart phone, or computer. They can also utilize speech generating devices (see **page 101**) such as laptop, and smartphone. Prior to the surgery it may be helpful to make a recording for one's answering machine or voicemail to inform callers about one's speaking difficulties.

An electrolarynx can be used to speak within a few days after the surgery. (See **Method of speaking section, Chapter 6, page 94**) Because of neck swelling and post-surgical stitches, the intra-oral route of delivering vibrations using a straw-like tube is preferred.

Long term survival

The prognosis of head and neck squamous cell carcinoma depends on the cancer's stage at diagnosis and its location. Survival rates represent the percentage of people who are alive within a certain period of time after treatment, but they should not be used to predict how cancer will affect a particular patient. Five-year overall survival in patients with stage I or stage II cancer is generally 70-90%. More advanced (stage III or IV) cancer and those who continue to smoke and consume alcohol have a poorer prognosis. Those with advanced laryngeal carcinoma have about 40 % five years survival.

The prognosis is better in HPV associated oropharyngeal cancers compared to non- HPV associated oropharyngeal cancers.

In general, the frequency of follow-up is greatest in the first two to four years following diagnosis because about 80 to 90% of all recurrences occur within this period. However, follow-up beyond five years is warranted because of the risks of late complications, late recurrence, and second malignancies. This is especially important for patients with non-HPV associated oropharyngeal cancers.

Pain management after surgery

The degree of pain experienced after laryngecomy (or any other head and neck surgery) is very subjective, but as a general rule, the more extensive the surgery, the more likely the patient will experience pain. Certain types of reconstructive procedures, where tissue is transferred as a flap from the chest muscles, forearm, thigh, jejunum, or a stomach pull up are more likely to be associated with increased or prolonged pain.

Those who have a radical neck dissection as part of the surgery may experience additional pain. At present, most patients undergo a "modified radical neck dissection" where the spinal accessory nerve is not removed. If the spinal accessory nerve is cut or removed during surgery, the patient is more likely to have shoulder discomfort, stiffness, and long term loss of range of motion. Some of the attendant discomfort of this procedure can be prevented by exercise and physical therapy.

For individuals who experience chronic pain as a result of laryngectomy or any other head and neck surgery, evaluation by a pain management specialist is usually very helpful.

Chapter 3:

Side effects of radiation treatment for head and neck cancer

RD is often used to treat head and neck cancer. It can be used as the only treatment, in combination with chemotherapy (chemoradiation therapy), or after surgery (adjuvant RT). The goal of RT is to kill cancer cells. Because these cells divide and grow at a faster rate than normal cells they are more likely to be destroyed by radiation. In contrast although they may be damaged, healthy cells generally recover.

Unfortunately RT causes short and long term side effects. RD can damage blood vessels that nourish muscles, nerves, and bones that can result in a progressive condition called "radiation fibrosis syndrome", which causes a variety of complications affecting nerve, muscles, and bones. (See **chapter 5, page 88**)

RT can be administered in several ways:

- *Organ preservation*-radiation is aimed at the tumor site (with or without chemotherapy) is used in an attempt to cure the disease without surgically removing the larynx. However, this is not always an option because of the size and location of the tumor and the recommendation is to proceed directly to surgery.
- *Palliative treatment-r*adiation (with or without chemotherapy) is given in an attempt to prolong life when the tumor is too large and/or inoperable and cure is highly unlikely.
- *Radiation after surgery-r*adiation is given after surgery to destroy any local residual cancer cells that may spread to other organs such as the lung, liver, or brain.
- *Reirradiation for recurrent cancer*-radiation is administered for recurrence of head and neck cancer in a previously irradiated area. Repeat irradiation with systemic therapy is a

potentially curative option. Long-term disease-free survival has been observed, albeit with the risk of significant, possibly life threatening, late complications.

Types of radiation therapy (RT)

Most patients with for head and neck cancers are treated with external beam RT (using X-rays or gamma rays). The current standard of care is to use intensity-modified RT (IMRT). This method adjusts the beams to maximize radiation to cancerous tissue and not to normal tissue. This reduces side effects of RT. An individual face mask is made for each patient to insure accurate delivery of radiation. The number of treatments a person may get depends on the cancer type. Some patients get radiation only a single time while others get radiation once a day, 5 days a week, for up to 7 weeks.

Other methods of radiation include:

- *Brachytherapy*-implanting radioactive source close to the cancer)
- *Intra-operative radiation therapy*
- *Neutron beam radiation therapy*-using higher energy neutron beams
- *Proton beam radiation therapy*-a more precise radiation
- *Radiosurgery*-using Cyberknife®, Gamma Knife® and LINAC
- *TomoTherapy*-combines precise 3-D imaging from computed tomography (CT) scanning with highly targeted radiation beams delivered precisely to the cancer while minimizing surrounding tissues damage
- *Conformal radiation therapy*-radiation beams are shaped to match the tumor's 3 dimensional picture based on CT and/or magnetic resonance imaging (MRI) scans
- *Radioactive iodine*-for thyroid cancer

If RT is recommended the radiation oncologist sets up a treatment plan that includes the total dose of radiation to be administered, the number of treatments to be given, and their schedule.

These are based on the type and location of the tumor, the patient's general health, and other present or past treatments. For early stage disease, doses of 66-74 Gy are generally administered.

The likelihood and severity of complications depends on a number of factors, including the total dose of radiation delivered, over what time it was delivered and what parts of the head and neck received radiation. The side effects of RT for head and neck cancer are divided into early (acute) and long term (chronic) effects. Early side effects occur during the course of therapy and during the immediate post therapy period (approximately 2-3 weeks after the completion of a course of RT). Late effects can manifest any time thereafter, from weeks to years later.

Patients are usually most bothered by the early effects of RT, although these will generally resolve over time. However, because long term effects may require lifelong care it is important to recognize these in order to prevent them and/or deal with their consequences. Knowledge of the radiation side effects can allow their early detection and proper management.

Individuals with head and neck cancer should receive counseling about the importance of smoking cessation. In addition to the fact that smoking is a major risk factor for head and neck cancer, the risk of cancer in smokers is further enhanced by alcohol consumption. Smoking can also influence cancer prognosis. When smoking is continued both during and after RT, it can increase the severity and duration of mucosal reactions, worsen the dry mouth (xerostomia), and compromise patient outcome. Patients who continue to smoke while receiving RT have a lower long-term survival rate than those who do not smoke.

1. Early side effects

Early side effects include inflammation of the oropharyngeal mucosa (mucositis), painful swallowing (odynophagia), difficulty swallowing (dysphagia), hoarseness, lack of saliva (xerostomia), orofacial pain, Laryngeal radionecrosis, dermatitis, hair loss, nausea, vomiting, inadequate nutrition and hydration, and weight loss. These complications can interfere with, and delay treatment. To some degree these side effects occur in most patients and generally dissipate over time.

The severity of these side effects is influenced by the amount and method by which the RT is given, the tumor's location and spread, and the patient's general health and habits (i.e. continued smoking, alcohol consumption).

Skin damage (radiation-induced dermatitis)

RT can cause a sunburn-like damage (radiation dermatitis) to the skin which can be further aggravated by chemotherapy. It is one of the most common side effects of RT and can cause pain and discomfort. The dermatitis depend upon the radiation dose and can be mild, moderate and severe. The severity of dermatitis and healing time are significantly increased in patients taking radiosensitizing agents.

It is advisable to keep the irradiated area clean and dry, wear loose-fitting clothes to avoid friction injuries, wash the skin with lukewarm water and mild soap (preferably synthetic soaps), and avoid exposure to potential chemical irritants, skin irritants such as perfumes and alcohol-based lotions, direct sun and wind, and local application of lotions or ointments prior to RT that might change the depth of radiation penetration.

There are a number of skin care products that can be used during RT to lubricate and protect the skin. These include aloe vera-based gels and water-based lotions. Although such preparations may provide symptom relief, none promotes or accelerates healing of the radiation-induced dermatitis.

Mild dermatitis starts improving with 10 days after completing of radiation, while severe dermatitis is associated with prolonged inflammation and healing time, resulting in skin fibrosis.

Skin cancer can rarely develop at the irradiated areas.

Wearing adhesive heat and moisture exchanger (HME) housing is not recommended during RT and the recovery period as the skin around the stoma usually become inflamed.

Hair loss

Hair follicles are very sensitive to radiation, and the treatments can cause hair loss. Most individuals observe hair loss within the treatment area about three weeks after the beginning RT. Hair loss may be temporary or permanent, depending on the total amount of radiation received and other treatments such as chemotherapy. When hair loss is temporary, it will likely re-grow within 3 to 6 months after treatment is complete. The re-growth of hair is often thinner or of a different texture.

Some individuals elect to have their hair cut short prior to starting RT. Those who wish to wear a wig, are advised to select it prior to losing their hair in order to match color and style.

The scalp is sensitive to radiation, especially following hair loss. The skin may become pink, tender or inflamed-like a sunburn. Following 2-3 weeks of treatment, the scalp may become dry and itchy. Appropriate special cream can be prescribed and applied to these areas.

The dry, irritated scalp is a temporary condition and start improving about two weeks after RT is complete. When indicated, medications can be administered to relieve discomfort and itching.

The scalp reaction can be minimized during the treatment by:

- Avoiding frequent shampooing and using a mild shampoo (such as baby shampoo) without any perfumes.
- Washing the scalp with warm water only and avoiding rubbing and scratching.
- Drying the washed area by patting with a dry soft towel.
- Avoiding excessively combing or brushing the hair.
- Avoiding the use of hair spray, oils or creams.

- Avoiding the use of heat sources (including hair dryers, rollers or curling irons).
- Avoiding perming or coloring the hair until about 4 weeks after RT is complete.
- Protecting the head from the sun, cold and wind by wearing a head covering (i.e., cap, scarf, and cotton hat).

Losing one's hair can be upsetting. Wearing a wig, scarves, turbans, bandanas, and hats having a short haircut can be helpful.

Dry mouth (xerostomia)

The loss of saliva production (or xerostomia) is the most common long-term complication of RT and is related to the administered irradiation dose and the volume of salivary tissue irradiated.

Prevention of permanent salivary gland damage can be attempted in selected patients by using parotid-sparing intensity-modulated radiation therapy (IMRT), reduce the radiation dose to the submandibular and minor salivary glands (if oncologically feasible), submandibular salivary gland surgical transfer, and administration of amifostine (a radiation protective organic thiophosphate medication).

Although xerostomia generally improves with time, it is often a permanent problem that can adversely impacts quality of life. Drinking adequate fluids, frequent sipping or spraying of the mouth with water; sucking on ice chips and /or sugar-free popsicles; and rinsing and gargling with a weak solution of salt and baking soda are helpful to refresh the mouth, loosen thick oral secretions, and alleviate mild pain.

The use of saliva substitutes, or stimulation of saliva production from intact salivary glandular tissues by taste/mastication, pharmacological sialogogues (a drug that increases the flow rate of saliva), acupuncture, avoiding all products that contain caffeine or alcohol, using a bedside humidifier at night, and raising the head of the bed can be helpful.

Soft and moistened foods, thick soups, mashed potatoes, puddings, and milkshakes are easier to eat and swallow.

For more information see Xerostomia at the **Late side effects** section **(page 54).**

Acceleration of periodontal disease

Patients who experience low function of their salivary gland and xerostomia must maintain excellent oral hygiene to minimize the risk of oral lesions.

Periodontal disease can be accelerated and caries can become rampant unless preventive measures are instituted. Multiple preventive strategies should be considered. This evolves performing systematic oral hygiene at least 4 times per day (after meals and at bedtime) which includes:

- Brushing teeth (if soreness of oral mucosa and trismus are present, a small ultra-soft toothbrush can be used).
- Using a fluoridated toothpaste when brushing
- If toothpaste makes one's mouth sore, brush with a solution of 1 teaspoon of salt mixed with 4 cups of water.
- Flossing once daily.
- Applying a prescription-strength fluoride gel at bedtime to prevent caries.
- Rinsing with a solution of salt and baking soda 4 to 6 times a day (½ tsp salt and ½ tsp baking soda in a cup of warm water) to clean and lubricate the oral tissues and to buffer the oral environment.
- Sipping water frequently to rinse the mouth and alleviate mouth dryness.
- Avoiding foods and liquids with a high sugar content.

Use of topical fluoride has demonstrable benefit in minimizing caries formation. It is recommended that during RT mouth guards be filled with topical 1% sodium fluoride gel and placed over the upper and lower teeth. The appliances should remain in place for 5 minutes, after which the patient should not eat or drink for 30 minutes.

Alterations in taste (dysgeusia)

Radiation can induce changes in taste as well as tongue pain. Foods can alternately taste too bland or too spicy due to the tongue's limited taste receptors. Some foods may taste different than they did in the past, some foods may taste bland, or every food may taste the same. Specifically, bitter, sweet, and salty foods may taste different, and some people may have a metallic or chemical taste in their mouth, especially after eating meat or other high-protein foods.

The sense of taste may also be affected by impaired smelling. These side effects can cause food aversion (dislike), further decrease food intake, and contribute to weight loss.

RT as well as chemotherapy can impair the sense of taste because of their effects on the in the tongue and nasal epithelium receptors. Additional factors that may contribute to an altered sense of taste include a bitter taste from chemotherapy drugs, poor oral hygiene, infection, and mucositis.

Taste changes and tongue pain caused by RT usually begin to improve three weeks to two months after the end of treatment. Improvement may continue for about a year, but the sense of taste may not entirely return to the way it was before treatment, especially if there is damage to the salivary glands.

In most instances, there are no specific treatments for taste problems.

These tips may help to cope with taste changes:

- Choosing foods that smell and taste good, even if the food is not familiar.

- Eliminating cooking smells by using an exhaust fan, cooking on an outdoor grill, or buying precooked foods. Cold or room-temperature foods also smell less.
- Eating cold or frozen food (i.e., frozen yogurt, ice cream), which may taste better than hot foods.
- Using plastic utensils and glass cookware to lessen a metallic taste.
- Trying sugar-free, mint gum or hard candies (with flavors such as mint, lemon, or orange) to mask a bitter or metallic taste in the mouth.
- Trying other protein sources (such as poultry, eggs, fish, peanut butter, beans, or dairy products) if red meats don't taste good.
- Marinating meats in fruit juices, sweet wines, salad dressings, or other sauces.
- Flavoring foods with herbs, spices, sugar, lemon, or sauces.
- Not eating one to two hours before and up to three hours after chemotherapy to prevent food aversions caused by nausea and vomiting. Additionally, avoiding favorite foods before chemotherapy helps prevent aversions to those foods.
- Rinsing with a salt and baking soda solution (½ teaspoon of salt and ½ teaspoon of baking soda in 1 cup of warm water) before meals, which may help neutralize bad tastes in the mouth.
- Keeping a clean and healthy mouth by brushing frequently and flossing daily.
- Considering zinc sulfate supplements, which may help improve taste in some people. However, one should consult with their physician before taking any dietary supplements, especially during active treatment.

Inflammation of the oropharyngeal mucosa (mucositis and odynophagia)

Radiation, as well as chemotherapy, damage the oropharyngeal mucosa resulting in mucositis, and odynophagia (pain with swallowing) which develops gradually, usually 2-3 weeks after starting RT. Its incidence and severity depend upon the field, total dose and duration of RT.

Chemotherapy can aggravate the condition. Mucositis can be painful and interfere with food intake and nutrition.

Management includes meticulous oral hygiene, dietary modification, and ingestion of topical anesthetics combined with an antacid and antifungal suspension ("cocktail") before eating. Spicy, acidic, sharp, or hot food, and alcohol should be avoided. Reducing the pain on swallowing can ease and increase food and liquid consumption. Secondary bacterial, viral (i.e., Herpes), and fungal (i.e., Candida or thrush) infections are possible. Control of the pain (using opiates or gabapentin) may be needed.

Currently, various strategies and agents have been described for the prevention of mucositis, including routine oral care, mucosal surface protectants, anti-inflammatory drugs, growth factors, certain antimicrobial formulations, laser therapy, oral cryotherapy, and specific natural and miscellaneous agents. These approaches encompass a diversity of mechanisms, but the results have been controversial, and the optimal prophylaxis remains unknown.

If toothpaste makes one's mouth sore, brushing with a solution of 1 teaspoon of salt mixed with 4 cups of water is less irritating.

Thrush prevention is described in the **Preventive care, Chapter 13 (page 199).**

Mucositis can lead to nutritional deficiency. Those who experience significant weight loss or recurrent episodes of dehydration may require feeding through a gastrostomy feeding tube.

When getting RT to the head or neck, one needs to take good care of their teeth, gums, mouth, and throat.

These tips may help one manage their mouth problems:

- Avoid spicy, sharp, crunchy and rough foods, such as raw vegetables, dry crackers, and nuts.
- Don't eat or drink very hot or very cold foods or beverages.
- Don't smoke, chew tobacco, or drink alcohol – these can make mouth sores worse.
- Stay away from sugary snacks.

- Ask your cancer care team to recommend a good mouthwash. The alcohol in some mouthwashes can dry and irritate mouth tissues.
- Avoid using toothpicks which can cut your mouth.
- If your gums are sore, only wear your dentures while eating.
- Rinse your mouth with warm salt and soda water every 1 to 2 hours as needed. (Use 1 teaspoon of salt and 1 teaspoon of baking soda in 1 quart of water.)
- Clean your mouth with a gauze square wrapped around your finger or a popsicle stick dipped in baking soda/salt rinse.
- Sip cool drinks often throughout the day.
- Eat sugar-free candy or chew gum to help keep your mouth moist.
- Moisten food with gravies and sauces to make it easier to eat.
- Clean your teeth and mouth after meals and before applying topical coating agents or medication for mouth sores.
- Use extra soft toothbrushes and soften them further by putting them in warm water. Change brushes often.
- If flavored toothpastes irritate your mouth, use plain baking soda.
- Ask your cancer care team about medicines to help treat mouth sores, and control pain while eating.

Viscid, copious mucus production is a major problem for many patients with severe mucositis. The mucus causes queasiness and gagging and contributes to difficulty in maintaining adequate hydration and nutrition.

The secretions can be managed by:

- Regular mouth rinsing with salt and soda solution, and taking oral guaifenesin in the early-phase of mucositis.
- Later-phase thickened or larger-volume mucus may respond to combination narcotics and anticholinergic drying agents present in some cough preparations.

- Treatment with mucus drying medications include: an antihistamine, and scopolamine transdermal patch.
- Elevation of the head of the patient's bed 30° can reduce edema and protect the airway.
- A cool mist vaporizer may help lubrication and expectoration.
- Lorazepam can help prevent repeated gagging and nausea.
- Suction machine can be useful, especially after surgery when effective gargle is difficult.

The duration of mucositis is proportional to the degree of mucosal stem cell depletion. Radiation-induced mucositis may take weeks to months to heal depending on mucosal stem cell recovery. Excessive depletion may prevent healing and lead to a chronic open wound recognized as "soft-tissue necrosis."

Laryngeal cartilage necrosis (Laryngeal radionecrosis)

Laryngeal radionecrosis (LR) is a rare complication following RT and is associated with significant morbidity and even mortality. One to 5% of patients undergoing radiotherapy may develop radiation-induced LR. Risk factors for the development of LR include smoking, tumor invasion, postoperative infection, trauma, and the radiation technique.

LR may develop at any time, shortly following treatment or even decades later. There are 5 grades of increasing severity of LR. Grades I and II are common post radiation changes and typically respond favorably to conservative treatment (i.e., humidification, voice restraint, discontinuation of smoking, antibiotics). Grade III and IV reactions are more severe, have less favorable outcomes, and are considered complications of radiotherapy. Severe LR is generally irreversible and often requires laryngectomy because of life-threatening laryngeal instability.

The typical patient with radiation-induced LR initially develops symptoms of hoarseness and breathiness. If airway distress develops, an emergent tracheotomy may be needed. If an individual has recurrent aspirations secondary to poor swallowing function, pneumonia and respiratory compromise can occur. Odynophagia and neck pain and stiffness are other late symptoms.

Pain in the mouth and/or face

Pain in the mouth and/or face (orofacial) is common in patients with head and neck cancer. It occurs in up to half of the patients before RT, 80% of patients during treatment and about one third of patients six months after treatment. The pain can be caused by mucositis which can be aggravated by concurrent chemotherapy, and by damage from the cancer, infection, inflammation, and scarring due to surgery or other treatments.

Pain management includes the use of analgesics and narcotics. Acupuncture can be used for pain and dry mouth after neck surgery and a dry mouth in individuals with advanced cancer.

Nausea and vomiting

RT may cause nausea. When it occurs, it generally happens from two to six hours after a RT session and lasts about two hours. Nausea may or may not be accompanied by vomiting. When feeling nausea breathing deeply and slowly and getting fresh air can help. Also distracting oneself with music or talking to a friend may help.

Management includes:

- Eating small, frequent meals throughout the day instead of three large meals. Nausea is often worse if one's stomach is empty

- Eating and drink slowly, chewing the food completely, and staying relaxed
- Eating cold or room temperature foods. The smell of warm or hot food may induce nausea
- Avoiding difficult to digest foods, such as spicy foods or foods high in fat or accompanied by rich sauces
- Avoiding nausea causing food
- Avoiding caffeine containing drinks and food
- Avoiding odors, perfumes, incense, and other strong smells
- Resting after eating. When lying down, the head should be elevated about 12 inches
- Drinking beverages and other fluids between meals instead of drinking beverages with meals
- Drinking 6-8 ounce glasses of fluid per day to prevent dehydration. Cold beverages, ice cubes, popsicle, or gelatin are adequate
- Eating more food at a time of the day when one is less nauseous
- Having someone else cook, as cooking may worsen nausea
- Informing one's health care provider before each treatment session when one develops persistent nausea
- Treating persistent vomiting immediately as this can cause dehydration
- Administering anti-nausea medication by a health care provider
- Wearing loose-fitted clothing can prevent irritation of one's throat or stomach and reduce nausea

Persistent vomiting can result in the body losing large amounts of water and nutrients. If vomiting persists for more than three times a day and one does not drink enough fluids, it could lead to dehydration. This condition can cause serious complications if left untreated.

Signs of dehydration include:

- Small amount of urine
- Dark urine

- Rapid heart rate

- Headaches

- Flushed, dry skin

- Coated tongue

- Irritability and confusion

Persistent vomiting may reduce the effectiveness of medications. If persistent vomiting continues, RT may be temporarily stopped. Fluids administered intravenously assist the body in regaining nutrients and electrolytes.

Difficult swallowing (dysphagia), inadequate nutrition and hydration

RT for head and neck cancer can cause many side effects that may contribute to inadequate calorie, protein and liquid intake. These side effects include lack of appetite, taste changes or lack of taste, painful chewing and swallowing (odynophagia), dry mouth, early satiety, diarrhea, nausea and general disinterest in food and eating.

It is important to continue to eat during RT. Not using the muscles of mastication weakens them. Furthermore, the scarring induced by radiation are reduced by chewing. Prophylactic swallowing exercises during chemotherapy and/or radiation can preserve normal swallowing. Exercises should address maintenance of strength and range of motion of the tongue/tongue base, pharyngeal constrictors, and the muscles responsible for hyolaryngeal excursion (hyoid bone and larynx move up) and airway protection. For those undergoing radiation following total laryngectomy, it is important to target tongue and tongue base strength. Jaw stretches are also an important part of treatment during radiation.

In addition to performance of swallowing exercises for prevention of radiation-associated dysphagia, maintaining oral intake during treatment has a positive impact on swallowing outcomes. The placement of a feeding tube is recommended only in high-risk patients or in response to nutritional deficiencies. Furthermore even when a tube is placed, the patient is encouraged to continue swallowing whatever is safe by mouth. The tube can provide supplemental nutrition but that the act of swallowing itself is a critical part of the treatment.

Calorie and protein needs are increased in individuals treated for cancer. These increased needs, combined with the many possible side effects, may lead to weight loss and dehydration. It is very important to try and maintain one's weight while receiving RT. It is advisable to obtain guidance from a dietitian how to maintain good nutrition and avoid weight loss and dehydration.

The basic principles to avoid weight loss and dehydration include:

- Eating small frequent meals-six to eight times per day
- Making every bite and sip count by eating calorie-dense foods and add calories to foods.
- Limiting foods and beverages low in calories
- Eating a variety of foods-include various colors, textures and flavors. Even though one needs a high calories and high protein diet, a balanced diet with foods from all food groups is essential. It is desirable to continue to include fruits and vegetables
- Carrying food at all times, to eat whenever possible
- Consuming liquid diet when swallowing becomes difficult. This can be prepared by using a blender or by ingesting bottled commercial food (i.e., Ensure, Boost)
- Consuming cold and/or frozen food (including ice cream) may be easier and can also reduce oral pain

As side effects worsen, most patients must focus on liquids and soft foods to obtain adequate calories. Often liquids can provide more calories than solids.

Selecting the best food is individual depending on taste and ability to swallow, and is often a trial and error process.

If ingestion of adequate calories and liquid is inadequate surgical installation of a gastric tube may be necessary. Placement of such a tube is also done prior to initiation of the RT to offer an alternative feeding route.

If dehydration and/or severe malnutrition occurs urgent admission to the hospital may be required to correct these.

Tiredness (fatigue)

Fatigue is one of the most common side effects of RT. RT can cause cumulative fatigue (fatigue that increases over time). It usually lasts from three to four weeks after treatment stops, but can continue for up to two to three months.

Fatigue can occur as the body repairs the damage to healthy cells and tissues. Some treatment side effects-such as anemia, pain, lack of sleep (insomnia) and rest, and changes in mood-also may cause fatigue.

Rest, energy conservation, and correcting the above contributing factors may ameliorate the fatigue.

The following strategies can reduce fatigue and improve the quality of life:

- Assess and document the level of fatigue daily by using a diary or worksheet to monitor fatigue daily. The fatigue level assessment includes monitoring its severity (none, minor, moderate, advanced) over the times the day.
- Perform regular daily tasks and activities especially during the time of day when feeling less fatigue. (Based upon one's diary or worksheet)
- Drink plenty of fluids and eat as nutritious as possible.
- Avoid caffeine which dries the mouth and can disrupt sleep.
- Maintain a daily exercise program.
- Allow plenty of time for sleep each night.

- Consult a social worker or a psychologist, and seek support from family and friends.
- Seek evaluation and treatment of underlying medical and psychological conditions (i.e., anemia, depression, hypothyroidism).
- Try to maintain a positive outlook.

Attention, thinking, and memory problems (cognitive problems)

Many patients who received RT to the head and neck and/or chemotherapy experience attention, thinking, or short-term memory problems (cognitive problems). Other causes for cognitive problems are pain, side effects of medications, emotional state, and other medical problems.

Cognitive problems can manifest in the following symptoms or behavioral changes:

- Trouble concentrating, focusing, or paying attention
- Mental fog or disorientation
- Difficulty with spatial orientation
- Memory loss or difficulty remembering things, especially names, dates, or phone numbers
- Problems with understanding
- Difficulties with judgment and reasoning
- Impaired ability to calculation and organize, and impaired language skills. These include difficulties to organize one's thoughts, find the right word, or balance a checkbook
- Problems in multitasking
- Processing information slower
- Behavioral and emotional changes, such as irrational behavior, mood swings, inappropriate anger or crying, and socially inappropriate behavior
- Severe confusion

Management of these cognitive problems includes:

- Medications, including stimulants, cognition-enhancing drugs, antidepressants, and drugs that block the actions of narcotics
- Occupational therapy and vocational rehabilitation, to help people with the activities of daily living and job-related skills
- Cognitive rehabilitation and cognitive training, to help patients improve their cognitive skills and find ways to cope with these issues.

Strategies for coping with cognitive problems include:

- Keeping a checklist of daily reminders
- Doing one task at a time without distractions
- Carrying around a small pad and a pen or pencil to write down notes and reminders. Or, downloading a note-making application on one's smartphone and tablet
- Using a calendar and a notebook with questions and a to-do list
- Letting friends, family, workplace, and health-care team know about one's memory loss
- Getting counseling and other resources to improve memory
- Placing sticky notes around the house and workplace as a reminder of important tasks
- Using word play, such as rhyming, to help you remember things
- Getting plenty of rest
- Keeping physically activity to increase mental alertness
- Conducting brain-strengthening mental activities (i.e., hobbies, solving puzzles, painting)
- Preparing for the next day by setting out the things one will need on the night before
- Color coding or labeling certain cabinets or drawers where one stores things around the home
- Eliminating clutter, and placing things back in the same place

Other side effects

These include trismus and hearing problems (see next section).

2. Late side effects

Late side effects include permanent loss of saliva; osteoradionecrosis; pharyngoesophageal stenosis; dental caries; oral cavity necrosis; fibrosis; impaired wound healing; skin changes and skin cancer; lymphedema; hypothyroidism; lightheadedness, dizziness and headaches; secondary cancer; and eye, ear, neurological and neck structures damage.

Permanent dry mouth (xerostomia)

Although the dry mouth (xerostomia) improves in most people with time, it can be long lasting and affects ones quality of life.

Saliva has important function that can be adversely affected following RT. These include:

- Lubrication and moistening of food for swallowing
- Solubilizing material so it can be tasted
- Initiating digestion
- Preventing dental caries
- Maintaining oral and upper gastrointestinal pH

- Health of oral mucosa
- Preventing opportunistic infections by maintaining oral microfloral balance
- Speech
- Denture / prosthesis comfort and function
- Cleansing of mouth and clearing the esophagus

RT can lead to irreversible salivary glands cell damage. Serous salivary glands (parotid & submandibular) are very sensitive to radiation. RT often leads to marked changes in the quantity and quality of saliva after just a few doses of radiation and alters the saliva's consistency from watery to more viscous.

Xerostomia can lead to:

- Opportunistic infections (mostly fungal such as thrush)
- Denture stomatitis
- Alterations in pH
- Alteration in secretory IgA
- Radiation caries (subgingival)

Aside from being bothersome to patients, by making it difficult to eat, swallow, and speak, there is greater risk of dental cavities and dental disease. The maintenance of dentures can also become problematic.

Patients who experience low function of their salivary gland and xerostomia must maintain excellent oral hygiene to minimize the risk of oral lesions. Periodontal disease can be accelerated and caries can become rampant unless preventive measures are instituted. Multiple preventive strategies should be considered.

Management and prevention include:

- Palliative use of salivary substitutes (gels; rinses)
- Non pharmacological saliva stimulation
- Salivary stimulants
- Prophylactic chlorhexidine
- Antifungal therapy
- Preventing thrush (see **Preventive care Chapter, page 199**)
- Drinking plenty of liquids

Management of xerostomia includes **salivary substitutes** or **artificial saliva** (containing hyetellose, hyprolose, or carmellose) and frequent sips of water. Increased water intake can lead to frequent urination especially at night in men with prostatic hypertrophy and in those with a small bladder. Other non-pharmacological substances that can stimulate salivary flow include acidic or bitter substances, and to a lesser degree sweet substances such as sugar-free hard candy. Chewing sugarless gum can provide both gustatory and tactile that increases salivary flow.

Available pharmacological medications include salivary stimulants (sialagogues), such as pilocarpine, amifostine, and cevimeline. Pilocarpine is the only drug approved by the U.S. Food and Drug Administration for use as a sialogogue for radiation xerostomia. Preliminary data suggest that hyperbaric oxygen can provides benefit for patients with xerostomia who have some residual salivary gland function. Acupuncture is widely used in Europe for a dry mouth in people having radiotherapy for head and neck cancers. It is also used for pain and dry mouth after neck surgery and a dry mouth in people with advanced cancer. Several clinical trials suggest that acupuncture can help.

Dietary change from dry, tough food to moist, softer one can greatly improve nutritional status and quality of life. Use of a humidification especially in the bedroom can also provide some relief.

Pharyngoesophageal stenosis

Pharyngoesophageal stenosis can be a delayed complication of RT. Pharyngoesophageal (PE) stenosis is an area of narrowing in the pharynx or esophagus. This stenosis can make it difficult to eat, particularly solid food. If the PE segment becomes completely closed off, the patient will not be able to eat or drink anything by mouth and will need a feeding tube placed directly into the stomach (gastric tube). Treatment of this complication might include frequent placement of dilating catheters down the throat to stretch open the narrowed segment or by surgically removing the blocked segment followed by flap reconstruction.

This is discussed in greater details in the **Swallowing difficulties** section in **Chapter 11 (page 168)**.

Dental caries

The risk of dental caries increases after RT for head and neck cancer because of a number of factors. These include increase in the number of caries producing bacteria (*Streptococcus mutans* and *Lactobacillus* species) in the mouth, reduced concentrations of salivary antimicrobial proteins, and loss of saliva's mineralizing components.

Treatment strategies must be directed to each component of the caries process. Optimal oral hygiene must be maintained and xerostomia should be managed whenever possible by using salivary substitutes or replacements. Caries resistance can be enhanced with the use of topical fluorides and/or remineralizing agents (high in calcium phosphate and fluoride). The efficacy of topical products may be enhanced by increasing their contact time with the teeth by using dental trays. Those unable to effectively comply with use of fluoride trays can be instructed to use brush-on gels and rinses.

Topical fluorides or chlorhexidine rinses may lead to reduced levels of *S. mutans* but not Lactobacilli. Because of adverse drug interactions, fluoride and chlorhexidine dosing should be separated by several hours.

Osteoradionecrosis of the jaw

This is one potentially severe complication that can necessitate surgical intervention and reconstruction. Depending on the location and extent of the lesion, symptoms may include pain, bad breath, taste distortion (dysgeusia), "bad sensation", numbness (anesthesia), trismus, difficulty with mastication and speech, fistula formation, pathologic fractures, and local, spreading, or systemic infection. Patients who have received high-dose radiation to the head and neck are at lifelong risk for osteoradionecrosis, with an overall risk of approximately 15%.

The jaw bone (mandible) is the most frequently affected bone, especially in those treated for nasopharyngeal cancer. Maxillary involvement is rare because of the collateral blood circulation it receives.

Tooth extraction and dental disease in irradiated areas are major factors in the development of osteoradionecrosis. In some cases it is necessary to remove teeth before RT if they will be in the area receiving radiation and are too decayed to preserve by filling or root canal. An unhealthy tooth can serve as a source of infection to the jaw bone that can be particularly difficult to treat after radiation.

Repair of nonrestorable and diseased teeth prior to RT may reduce the risk of this complication. Oral disease should be eliminated pretreatment whenever possible. Dentition that exhibits poor prognosis and is within high-dose radiation fields should be extracted before RT begins. Ideally, at least 7 to 14 days should be allowed for healing before initiation of RT; some have suggested allowing up to 21 days.

Mild osteoradionecrosis can be conservatively treated with debridement, antibiotics, and occasionally ultrasound. Topical antibiotics (e.g., tetracycline) or antiseptics (e.g., chlorhexidine) may contribute to wound resolution. Wherever possible, exposed bone should be covered with mucosa and necrotic bone removed. Analgesics for pain control are often effective. When necrosis is extensive, radical resection, followed by microvascular reconstruction is often used.

Hyperbaric oxygen therapy (HBO) has been often used in patients at risk or those who develop osteoradionecrosis of the jaw (See **Chapter 14, page 207).** However, the available data are conflicting about the clinical benefit of HBO for prevention and therapy of osteoradionecrosis.

HBO has been reported to increase oxygenation of irradiated tissue, promote angiogenesis, and enhance osteoblast repopulation and fibroblast function. HBO is usually prescribed as 20 to 30 dives at 100% oxygen and 2 to 2.5 atmospheres of pressure. If surgery is needed, ten dives of postsurgical HBO are recommended. Unfortunately, HBO technology is not always accessible to patients who might otherwise benefit because of lack of available units and the high price of care.

Patients should inform their dentists about their RT prior to extraction or dental surgery. Osteonecrosis may be prevented by administration of a series of HBO therapy before and after these procedures. This is recommended if the involved tooth is in an area that has been exposed to a high dose of radiation. Consulting the radiation oncologist who delivered the RT can be helpful in determining the extent of prior exposure.

Dental prophylaxis can reduce the risk of osteoradionecrosis. Special fluoride treatments may help with dental problems along with brushing, flossing, and regular cleaning by a dental hygienist.

A home care dental lifelong routine is recommended:

1. Flossing each tooth and brushing with toothpaste after each meal.

2. Brushing the tongue with a tongue brush or a soft bristled toothbrush once a day.

3. Rinsing with a baking soda rinse daily. Baking soda helps neutralize the mouth. One teaspoon added to 12 oz. of water. The baking soda rinse can be used throughout the day.

4. Using fluoride in fluoride carriers once a day. Fluoride carriers are custom made by a professional dentist. A 1.1% sodium fluoride or 0.4% stannous fluoride is placed in the

fluoride carriers and applied over the teeth for 10 minutes. One should not rinse, drink, or eat for 30 minutes after fluoride application.

Necrosis in the oral cavity

Tissue necrosis (death of cells) and secondary infection of previously irradiated tissue is a serious complication for patients who have undergone RT for head and neck cancer. Acute damage typically involves the mucosa of the mouth. Chronic changes involving bone and mucosa are a result of the process of vascular inflammation and scarring that results in tissue damage because of reduced blood and oxygen supply. Infection secondary to tissue injury and osteonecrosis confounds the process (see **page 58**).

Soft tissue necrosis can occur in any mucosal surface in the mouth. Trauma and injury are often associated with nonhealing soft tissue necrotic lesions, though spontaneous lesions can also happen. Soft tissue necrosis begins as an ulcerative break in the mucosal surface and can spread in diameter and depth. Pain will generally become more prominent as soft tissue necrosis becomes worse. Secondary infection can also take place.

Excessive depletion may prevent healing and lead to a chronic open wound recognized as *soft-tissue necrosis*. This may be referred to as a *consequential late effect*. Other consequential late effects include mucosal scarring (healing by secondary intention) and loss of mucosal compliance, contributing to chronic dysphagia.

Fibrosis and trismus

High doses of radiation to the head and neck can result in fibrosis. This condition may be aggravated after head and neck surgery where the neck may develop a woody texture and have limited movement. Radiation-induced fibrosis can develop as a late effect of RT in skin and subcutaneous tissue, muscles, or other organs, depending upon the treatment site. Radiation-induced fibrosis may cause both cosmetic and functional impairment, which can lead to deterioration in the quality of life.

Late onset of fibrosis can also occur in the pharynx and esophagus, leading to stricture and temporomandibular joint problems including mandibular dysfunction. Patients can be instructed in physical therapy interventions such as mandibular stretching exercises and the use of prosthetic aids designed to reduce the severity of fibrosis. It is important that these approaches be instituted before trismus develops. If clinically significant changes develop, several approaches can be considered, including stabilization of occlusion, and use of trigger-point injection and other pain management strategies, muscle relaxants, and tricyclic medications.

Fibrosis of the muscles of mastication can lead to the inability to open the mouth (**trismus or lockjaw**) which can progress over time. The prevalence of trismus increases with increasing doses of radiation, and levels in excess of 60 Gy are more likely to cause trismus. Generally, eating becomes more difficult but articulation is not affected. Radiation of the highly vascularized temporomandibular joint (TMJ) and muscles of mastication can often lead to trismus. Chronic trismus gradually leads to fibrosis.

Trismus impedes proper oral care and treatment and may cause speech/swallowing deficits. Forced opening of the mouth, jaw exercises and the use of a dynamic opening device (Therabite ™) can be helpful. This device is increasingly used during RT as a prophylactic measure to prevent trismus. One of the benefits of the Therabite System is that it not only stretches the connective tissue that causes trismus, but also allows for proper mobilization of the temporomandibular joint, thus addressing a secondary cause of pain and tightness.

Early treatment of trismus has the potential to prevent or minimize many of the consequences of this condition. As restriction becomes more severe and likely irreversible, the need for treatment becomes more urgent.

A wide array of appliances are available for the **treatment of trismus**. Devices range widely in cost. Many devices must be custom made for each patient, thus increasing the cost of treatment. Others, such as continuous passive motion devices are rented on a daily or weekly basis.

These devices include the following:

- Cages that fit over the head
- Heavy springs that fit between the teeth
- Screws that are placed between the central incisors
- Hydraulic bulbs placed between the teeth
- The most commonly used treatment is the use of tongue depressors. These are stacked, forced and held between the teeth in an attempt to push the mouth open over time

Muscle tightness can often serve as trigger of **headaches** which may eventually lead to migraine. Treatment of muscle fibrosis can often alleviate and reduce the frequency of such headaches.(See **page 62**)

Exercise can reduce neck tightness and increases the range of neck motion. One needs to perform these exercises throughout life to maintain good neck mobility. This is especially the case if the stiffness is due to radiation. Receiving treatment by experienced physical therapies who can also break down the fibrosis is very helpful. The earlier the intervention, the better it is for the patient. There are physical therapy experts in most communities who specialize in reducing swelling.

Fibrosis in the head and neck can become even more extensive in those who have had surgery or further radiation. Post radiation fibrosis can also involve the skin and subcutaneous tissues, causing discomfort and lymphedema.

A new treatment modality that reduces lymphedema, fibrosis and neck muscle stiffness using **external laser** is also available. This method uses a low energy laser beam administered by an experienced physical therapist. The laser beam penetrates the tissues where it is absorbed by cells and changes their metabolic processes. The beam is generated by the LTU-904 Portable Laser Therapeutic Unit.

Swallowing dysfunction due to fibrosis often requires a change in diet, pharyngeal strengthening, or swallow retraining, especially in those who have had surgery and/or chemotherapy. Swallowing exercises are increasingly used as a preventing measure.

Partial or total oropharyngeal stricture can occur in severe cases. (See **Chapter 11, Narrowing of the neopharynx and esophagus Section, page 171**)

Impaired wound healing

Some patients may manifest wound healing impairment following surgery, especially in areas that have received RT. Some may develop a fistula (an abnormal connection between the inside of the throat and the skin). (See **Chapter 11, page 177**). Wounds that heal at a slower pace can be treated with antibiotics and dressing changes by specialists.

Skin changes and skin cancer

Patients who suffered from an initial severe dermatitis, may experience inflammatory waves that can occur weeks to years after their RT. Late-stage or chronic radiation dermatitis typically presents months to years after radiation exposure. It is characterized by skin fibrosis, slight color changes to the skin or mild swelling, atrophy, and widened blood vessels on the skin (telangiectasias).

Patients treated with RT can experience radiation recall dermatitis. Its estimated frequency is in 9% of individuals. Symptoms of radiation recall are induced by inflammation in a region that was previously treated with radiation. The reaction is characterized by a skin rash typified by redness, swelling, and/or blistering of the skin. The rash is often painful and can resemble a severe sunburn. (See **Chapter 3, Early side effects of radiation section, page 38**)

Individuals generally lose hair in the region that received radiation (see above).

Radiation can increase the risk for skin cancers in the area that received radiation. The most common types of skin cancers seen are basal cell carcinoma and squamous cell carcinoma. Therefore, it is very important to see a dermatologist regularly. When noticing any changes in the texture or color of the skin in the radiated area or any new lesions in the field, one should bring those to the attention of their health care providers for further evaluation.

Lymphedema

Obstruction of the cutaneous lymphatics results in lymphedema. Significant pharyngeal or laryngeal edema may interfere with breathing and may require temporary or long term tracheostomy. Lymphedema, strictures, and other dysfunctions predispose patients to aspiration and the need for a feeding tube. (See **Lymphedema, Chapter 5, page 84**)

Hypothyroidism

RT is almost always associated with hypothyroidism. The incidence varies; it is dose-dependent and increases as time elapsed since the RT. (See **Hypothyroidism, Chapter 12, page 186**)

Neurological damage

RT to the neck can also affect the spinal cord, resulting in a self-limited transverse myelitis, known as "Lhermitte's sign". The patient notes an electric shock-like sensation mostly felt with neck bending (flexion). This condition rarely progresses to a true transverse myelitis which is associated with Brown-Séquard syndrome (A loss of sensation and motor function caused by the lateral cutting of the spinal cord) and typically resolves within one year.

RT may cause neuropathy due to nerve injury, although it may take several years for symptoms to appear. RT can also cause peripheral nervous system dysfunction resulting from external compressive fibrosis of soft tissues and reduced blood supply caused by fibrosis. Peripheral neuropathy (see **Chapter 4**, **Side effects of chemotherapy for head and neck cancer** section, **page 79**) is a disorder that occurs when the nerves outside the brain and spinal cord, called the peripheral nervous system, are damaged. Depending on which nerves are affected, symptoms that include a change in sensation, especially in the hands and feet, (e.g., numbness, tingling, or pain), muscle weakness, (i.e., myopathy), and changes in organ function (i.e., constipation, dizziness) can occur.

Acupuncture treatment may improve peripheral neuropathy.

Damage to the peripheral and autonomic nervous system can lead to dizziness when standing up from sitting up from sitting or lying down due to **postural hypotension**.

RT of head and neck cancer seemed to have adverse but insignificant effects on the cognitive functions of the patients.

Eye damage

Cataract: Radiation can cause cataract usually in the posterior sub-capsular and sometimes in the cortical areas of the lens. It is important to note that many other confounding risk factors contribute to lens opacities which include age, diabetes mellitus, corticosteroids use, smoking, and ultraviolet radiation exposure. Although much work has been carried out in this area, the exact mechanisms of how radiation causes cataract are still not fully understood.

A number of studies indicate that there is risk of lens opacities at doses below 1 Gy and the threshold may range from none to 0.8 Gy. However, the International Commission on Radiological Protection has recently accepted the threshold of 0.5 Gy.

Many years or decades could pass before radiation-induced eye lens injuries become apparent. At relatively high exposures of few Gy, lens opacities may occur within a few years; however, at lower doses and dose rates (<1 Gy), lens opacities may occur after many years. The duration of the latency period is inversely dependent on dose.

The only way to treat cataract is by surgery. This involves removing the opacified lens, leaving the capsule that contains it intact. A plastic lens is inserted and, therefore, there is no need to wear special glasses after the operation. Surgery is only indicated when lens opacity progresses to a stage that causes visual disability.

Radiation retinopathy: Radiation retinopathy is a complication following exposure to any source of radiation. It is especially common after RT for nasopharyngeal, paranasal sinus or orbital tumors. Higher total radiation dose has been shown to increase the risk of radiation retinopathy. The incidence of retinopathy increases at doses above 45 Gy.

Comorbidities such as diabetes, hypertension, simultaneous chemotherapy and pregnancy are associated with an increased risk of radiation retinopathy.

Appropriate shielding of the ocular structures during external beam radiation and hyperfractionation of external beam can decreased the incidence of radiation retinopathy.

Patients with early or mild retinopathy may be asymptomatic. Other patients with more advanced disease can present with decreased vision or floaters.

Treatment includes intravitreal injection of humanized monoclonal antibody to vascular endothelial growth factor (Bevacizumab), intravitreal triamcinolone acetonide, grid macular laser photocoagulation, sector scatter and pan-retinal laser photocoagulation, photodynamic therapy, hyperbaric oxygen and oral pentoxifylline. Advanced proliferative radiation retinopathy complicated by vitreous hemorrhage and/or tractional retinal detachment may require vitrectomy.

Damage to the ear (ototoxicity) and hearing loss

Common complaints experienced by the patients after RT are ear heaviness, earache, decreased hearing, tinnitus, and dizziness. Patients who undergo RT for head and neck cancer appear more likely to experience hearing loss and to be more disabled by its effects than those who do not receive such treatment. Dose of radiation is directly proportional to ototoxicity; minimum 60 Gys of total radiation dose is required to produce significant ototoxicity.

Chemoradiation therapy can cause progressive hearing impairment especially in those receiving the chemotherapy intravenously, with a modest deterioration of 5 decibel 4.5 years after treatment.

Radiation to the ear may result in serous otitis (otitis with effusion). This is a condition associated with accumulation of fluid in the middle ear and a temporary reduced hearing. This condition and conductive deafness are reversible over time. High doses of radiation can cause and sensorineural hearing loss (damage to the inner ear, the auditory nerve, or the vestibular apparatus).This condition is not reversible. Damage to the vestibular apparatus can cause dizziness and vertigo.

Lightheadedness, dizziness and headaches

Lightheadedness, dizziness, and headaches can be one of a late side effects of radiation of the head and neck. Damage to the peripheral and autonomic nervous system can lead to dizziness when standing up from a sitting or lying down, due to the development of low blood pressure (orthostatic hypotension). This can be prevented by standing up slowly, wearing of compression stockings, exercises and by keeping well hydrated. It is best to consult one's physician to prevent and treat this condition.

The perception of the body's position is determined by the brain by integrating information from the middle ear, eyes, and the body's muscles and joints. Unfortunately, radiation almost always causes head neck muscles fibrosis and can also infrequently damage the middle ear. The perception of lightheadedness and dizziness after RT may be generated in some individuals by misinformation sent to the cerebellum (the part of the brain that controls the body's balance) which is inaccurate and contradictory.

Dizziness and lightheadedness can be treated by physical therapy. This includes vestibular rehabilitation and exercises that stretch the fibrotic muscles, reduce neck stiffness, and increase the head and neck range of motion. One needs to perform these exercises throughout life to maintain good neck mobility.

Vestibular rehabilitation therapy is an exercise-based program designed to promote central nervous system compensation for inner ear deficits as well as misinformation sent to the brain from other parts of the body (eyes, skin, muscle, joints, etc.).

Dizziness and lightheadedness can be caused by a variety of causes and conditions and should be evaluated by one's physician and medical specialists (e.g., neurologist, otolaryngologist).

Muscle tightness and fibrosis can often serve as trigger of headaches which may eventually lead to migraine. Treatment of muscle fibrosis can often alleviate and reduce the frequency of such headaches.

Damage to neck structures

Neck edema and fibrosis are common after RT. Over time the edema may harden, leading to neck stiffness. Damage can also include carotid artery narrowing (stenosis) and stroke, carotid artery rupture, oropharyngo-cutaneous fistula (the last two are associated also with surgery), and carotid artery baroreceptors damage leading to permanent and proxysmal (sudden and recurrent) hypertension.

Carotid artery stenosis and carotid artery rupture: The carotid arteries (CA) in the neck supply blood to the brain. Radiation to the neck has been linked to CA stenosis or narrowing, and rarely to CA rupture; representing a significant risk for head and neck cancer patients, including laryngectomees. Screening ultrasound within the first year since completion of radiotherapy, followed by repeat ultrasounds every two to three years and whenever CA stenosis is suspected can lead to early diagnosis. Smoking increases the risk of CA stenosis. The cumulative risk of stroke after RT is 12%. CA disease can cause strokes and transient ischemic attack (TIA), though it does not always cause symptoms. It is important to diagnose carotid stenosis or impending rupture early, before a stroke or severe bleeding has occurred.

Stenosis can be diagnosed by ultrasound as well as angiography. Treatment includes removal of the blockage (endarterectomy), placing a stent (a small device placed inside the artery to widen it) or a prosthetic carotid bypass grafting.

Evidence suggesting impending rupture can be obtained on physical and radiological examinations. Endovascular stenting is also performed in patients with impending carotid artery rupture.

Hypertension due to baroreceptors damage: Radiation to the head and neck can damage the baroreceptors located in the carotid artery. These baroreceptors help in regulating blood pressure by detecting the pressure of blood flowing through them, and sending messages to the central nervous system to increase or decrease the peripheral vascular resistance and cardiac output. Some individual treated with radiation develop labile or paroxysmal hypertension.

Labile hypertension: In this condition the blood pressure fluctuates far more than usual within the day. It can rapidly soar from low (e.g., 120/80 mm Hg) to high (e.g., 170/105 mm Hg). In many instances these fluctuations are asymptomatic but may be associated with headaches. A relationship between blood pressure elevation and stress or emotional distress is usually present.

Paroxysmal hypertension: Patients exhibit sudden elevation of blood pressure (which can be greater than 200/110 mm Hg) associated with an abrupt onset of distressful physical symptoms, such as headache, chest pain, dizziness, nausea, palpitations, flushing, and sweating. Episodes can last from 10 minutes to several hours and may occur once every few months to once or twice daily. Between episodes, the blood pressure is normal or may be mildly elevated. Patients generally cannot identify obvious psychological factors that cause the paroxysms. Medical conditions that can also cause such blood pressure swings need to be excluded (e.g., pheochromocytoma).

Both of these conditions are serious and should be treated. Management can be difficult and should be done by experienced specialists.

Secondary cancers

Even though radiation is used to treat cancer, paradoxically, years later it can rarely result in new local and systemic cancers appearing. The risk increases with high dosage and greater time since treatment. The secondary cancer can be quite different from the original and could include local cancers such as skin, mediastinal, oral and thyroid cancer, and systemic cancers such as lymphomas, sarcomas and leukemia. It is important to be closely followed by one's physician as well as medical specialists (i.e., dermatologist) to detect secondary malignancies.

More information about complications of RT can be found at the National Cancer Institute Web site https://www.cancer.gov/about-cancer/treatment/side-effects/mouth-throat/oral-complications-pdq#section/all

Chapter 4:

Side effects of chemotherapy for head and neck cancer

Chemotherapy for head and neck cancer is used in conjunction with supportive care for most patients with metastatic or advanced recurrent head and neck cancer. The choice of specific systemic therapy is influenced by the patient's prior treatment with chemotherapeutic agents and the general approach to preserve the affected organs. Supportive care includes the prevention of infection due to severe bone marrow suppression and the maintenance of adequate nutrition.

There are many different types of chemotherapy medications that differ in how they kill the cancer cells. The choice of agents(s) is based on clinical trials that have shown which ones are effective. Therapeutic options include treatment with a single agent and combination regimens with conventional cytotoxic chemotherapy and/or molecularly targeted agents, combined with optimal supportive care. Chemotherapy is given in cycles, alternating between periods of treatment and rest. Treatment can last several months or even longer.

The agents commonly used in treatment head and neck cancer include: Cisplatin, carboplatin, 5-fluorouracil, hydroxyurea, paclitaxel and docetaxel, and epirubicin. Other less commonly agents include: gemcitabine, vinorelbine and irinotecan, methotrexate and edatrexate, and ifosfamide. Cetuximab, vandetanib, trametinib and bevacizumab, are newer drug that target a specific receptor molecule that is found on some head and neck cancer cells. Enclosed is a link to a site that lists all the chemotherapeutic agents and their side effects.

https://stanfordhealthcare.org/medical-treatments/c/chemotherapy/side-effects/drugs-side-effects.html

Chemotherapeutic drugs work throughout the whole body by disrupting cancer cells' growth. The drugs can be given intravenously (most common), intra-muscularly, and by mouth. Chemotherapy for the treatment of head and neck cancers is usually given at the same time as

RT and is known as chemoradiation. It can be given as adjuvant chemotherapy or as neoadjuvant chemotherapy.

Adjuvant chemotherapy is used for treatment after surgery to reduce the risk of cancer returning, and to kill cells that may have spread. *Neoadjuvant chemotherapy* is administered before surgery to shrink the size of the tumor thus making it easier to remove. Chemotherapy administered prior to chemoradiation treatment is known as *induction chemotherapy.*

Side effects of chemotherapy

The kind and type of possible side effects of chemotherapy depend on the individual. Some have few side effects, while others have more. Many individuals do not experience side effects until the end of their treatments; for many individuals, these side effects do not last long. Chemotherapy can, however, cause several temporary and long term side effects. Although these may be worse with combined radiation therapy (RT), they generally disappear gradually after the treatment has ended.

Side effects depend on the chemotherapeutic agent(s) used. These occur because chemotherapy drugs work by killing all actively growing cells. These include cells of the digestive tract, hair follicles, and bone marrow (which makes red and white blood cells), as well as the cancer cells.

The more common side effects are nausea, vomiting, taste alteration, diarrhea, sores (mucositis) in the mouth (resulting in problems swallowing and sensitivity in the mouth and throat), increased susceptibility to infection, anemia, hair loss, general fatigue, numbness in the hands and feet (neuropathy), hearing loss, kidney damage, radiation recall dermatitis, bleeding problems, malaise, and balance problem. An oncologist and other medical specialist watch for and treat these side effects.

Lowered resistance to infection

Chemotherapy can temporarily reduce the production of white blood cells (neutropenia), making the patient more susceptible to infections.

This effect may begin about seven days following treatment and the decline in resistance to infection is maximal usually about 10–14 days after chemotherapy has ended. At that point the blood cells generally begin to increase steadily and return to normal before the next cycle of chemotherapy is administered. Signs of infection include fever above 100.4°F (38°C) and or a sudden feeling of being ill. Prior to resuming chemotherapy blood test are performed to ensure the recovery of the white blood cells has occurred. Further administration of chemotherapy may be delayed until recovery of blood cells has taken place.

Bruising or bleeding

Chemotherapy can promote bruising or bleeding because the agents given reduce the production of platelets which help the blood clotting. Nosebleeds, blood spots or rashes on the skin, and bleeding gums can be a sign that this has occurred.

Anemia

Chemotherapy can lead to anemia (low number of red blood cells). The patient generally feels tired and breathless. Severe anemia can be treated by blood transfusions or medications that promote red cells production.

Kidney problems (nephropathy)

A variety of renal disease can be caused by many chemotherapeutic agents. These agents can affect the glomerulus, tubules, and the interstitium of the kidney. Individuals can exhibit a variety of clinical manifestations ranging from an asymptomatic increase of their serum creatinine to acute renal failure requiring dialysis.

Hair loss

Some chemotherapy agents cause hair loss all over the body. The hair almost always grows back over a period of 3-6 months once the chemotherapy has ended. Meanwhile, a wig, bandana, hat or scarf can be worn.

These steps can minimize the frustration and anxiety associated with hair loss:

Before treatment:

- Do not bleach, color or perm the hair
- Do not dry the hair with heating devices such as curling irons and hot rollers.
- Considering cutting or shortening the. Short hair tends to look fuller than long hair.
- Plan for a wig, scarves or other head coverings. The cost of a wig may be covered by health insurance if one's doctor writes a prescription for it.

During treatment:

- Use a soft brush
- Wash your hair only as often as necessary with a gentle shampoo.
- Consider shaving the head. Some people report that their scalps feel itchy, sensitive and irritated during their treatments and while their hair is falling out. Shaving the head can

reduce the irritation and save the embarrassment of shedding. Some men shave their heads because they feel it looks better than the patchy hair loss they might be experiencing.

- Protecting the scalp from to the sun or to cold air, with sunscreen or a head covering. The scalp may be sensitive during the treatment, and extreme cold or sunshine can easily irritate it.

After treatment:

- Continue gentle hair care as the new hair growth is fragile and vulnerable to the damage caused by styling products and heating devices.
- Hold off on coloring or bleaching until the hair grows stronger. Processing could damage the new hair and irritate the sensitive scalp.
- Be patient. The hair may come back slowly and might not look normal right away. Growth takes time, and it takes time to repair the damage caused by the cancer treatment.

Hearing loss

Hearing loss is a special common for platinum-based chemotherapy drugs (i.e., cisplatin). Associated symptoms my include ringing in the ears (tinnitus). The hearing loss begins in the upper hearing frequencies; often well above the range for speech recognition. The patient often doesn't realize that the damage has begun until ototoxicity has irrevocably impacted the cochlear hair cells and other critical parts of the inner ear.

Chemoradiation therapy can cause progressive hearing impairment especially in those receiving the chemotherapy intravenously, with an average of 5 decibel decrease in hearing 4.5 years after treatment. It is advisable that patients have a hearing test prior to treatment with a platinum-based chemotherapy, followed by repeated tests throughout their treatment.

Sore mouth (mucositis), thrush and small mouth ulcers

Some chemotherapeutic agents cause sore mouth (mucositis) which can interfere with mastication and swallowing, oral bleeding, difficulty in swallowing (dysphagia), dehydration, heartburn, vomiting, nausea, and sensitivity to salty, spicy, and hot/cold foods. These agents can also cause chemotherapy-related oral cavity ulcers (stomatitis), and thrush that result in eating difficulty.

The cytotoxic agents most often associated with oral, pharyngeal, and esophageal symptoms of swallowing difficulty (dysphagia) are the antimetabolites such as methotrexate and fluorouracil. The radiosensitizer chemotherapies, designed to heighten the effects of RT, also increase the side effects of the radiation mucositis (See **Chapter 3, page 43**).

Nausea and vomiting can be treated by anti-nausea (anti-emetic) drugs. Regular mouthwashes can also help. These side effects can impact swallowing and nutrition. Accordingly, it is important to supplement one's diet with nutritious drinks or soups. A dietitian's advice may be helpful to maintain adequate nutrition. Mucositis can lead to nutritional deficiency. Those who experience significant weight loss or recurrent episodes of dehydration may require feeding through a gastrostomy feeding tube.

Management includes meticulous oral hygiene, dietary modification, and topical anesthetics combined with an antacid and antifungal suspension ("cocktail"). Spicy, acidic, sharp, or hot food as well as alcohol should be avoided. Secondary bacterial, viral (i.e., Herpes), and fungal (i.e., Candida) infections are possible. Control of the pain (using opiates or gabapentin) may be needed.

Prevention and treatment of thrush can be found in the **Preventive care** chapter (**Chapter 13, page 199**).

Alterations in taste (dysgeusia)

Chemotherapy as well as RT can impair the sense of taste because of their effects on the in the tongue and nasal epithelium receptors. Additional factors that may contribute to an altered sense of taste include a bitter taste from chemotherapy drugs, poor oral hygiene, infection, and mucositis. These side effects can further decrease food intake and contribute to weight loss.

The altered taste and tongue pain gradually dissipate in most patients over a six month period, although in some cases taste recovery is incomplete. Many individuals experience a permanent alteration in their taste.

In most instances, there are no specific treatments for taste problems.

These tips may help to cope with taste changes:

- Choosing foods that smell and taste good, even if the food is not familiar.
- Eliminating cooking smells by using an exhaust fan, cooking on an outdoor grill, or buying precooked foods. Cold or room-temperature foods also smell less.
- Eating cold or frozen food, which may taste better than hot foods. This is not the case in those receiving oxaliplatin (Eloxatin), which makes it difficult to ingest anything cold.
- Using plastic utensils and glass cookware to lessen a metallic taste.
- Trying sugar-free, mint gum or hard candies (with flavors such as mint, lemon, or orange) to mask a bitter or metallic taste in the mouth.
- Trying other protein sources (such as poultry, eggs, fish, peanut butter, beans, or dairy products) if red meats don't taste good.
- Marinating meats in fruit juices, sweet wines, salad dressings, or other sauces.
- Flavoring foods with herbs, spices, sugar, lemon, or sauces.
- Not eating one to two hours before and up to three hours after chemotherapy to prevent food aversions caused by nausea and vomiting. Additionally, avoiding favorite foods before chemotherapy helps prevent aversions to those foods.

- Rinsing with a salt and baking soda solution (½ teaspoon of salt and ½ teaspoon of baking soda in 1 cup of warm water) before meals, which may help neutralize bad tastes in the mouth.

- Keeping a clean and healthy mouth by brushing frequently and flossing daily.

- Considering zinc sulfate supplements, which may help improve taste in some people. However, one should consult with their physician before taking any dietary supplements, especially during active treatment.

Nausea and vomiting

Chemotherapy-induced nausea and vomiting (CINV) may be very distressing. CINV is a common problem with all chemotherapeutic agents. It can be acute (beginning within 1-2 hours of chemotherapy, peaking in 4-6 hours); delayed (beginning within 24 hours); chronic and anticipatory (occurring prior to treatment).

There are available therapeutic modalities that include medications and acupuncture aimed at the prevention and treatment of CINV. Acupuncture can be used to help relieve nausea) caused by chemotherapy or other cancer drugs. Seabands (acubands) are bracelets that apply pressure to acupuncture points on the wrist and can help to reduce sickness due to chemotherapy or following surgery.

Radiation recall dermatitis

"Radiation recall"-also called "radiation recall dermatitis"-is an inflammatory reaction that occurs when an individual receives chemotherapy following RT for cancer. Its estimated frequency is in 9% of individuals. Symptoms of radiation recall are induced by inflammation in a region that was previously treated with radiation. The reaction is characterized by a skin rash typified by redness, swelling, and/or blistering of the skin. The rash is often painful and can resemble a severe sunburn.

The chemotherapy agents most commonly associated with radiation recall include: Docetaxel (Taxotere), Paclitaxel (Taxol), Gemcitabine (Gemzar), Capecitabine (Xeloda), and Doxorubicin (Adriamycin).

Treatment for the reaction is mostly supportive, initially by eliminating the source of the reaction (i.e., discontinuing the responsible chemotherapy drug). Medications such as corticosteroids and anti-inflammatory agents may be used.

Unfortunately, it is difficult to predict who will react to a particular chemotherapy drug following RT. Radiation recall occurs less often when the time interval between the RT and chemotherapy is longer. However, considerations other than radiation recall are often more important in making decisions about timing of chemotherapy treatments.

Chemotherapy-induced peripheral neuropathy

Disorders of peripheral nerves are frequent complications of chemotherapy. Chemotherapy can cause degeneration of peripheral sensory and motor nerves and cause patients to present with sensory disturbances, balance problems or weakness.

Specific types of chemotherapeutic agents, particularly in high doses, can injure peripheral nerves. These drugs include: Bortezomib (Velcade); Platinums, including cisplatin (Platinol), oxaliplatin (Eloxatin), and carboplatin (Paraplatin); Taxanes, including docetaxel (Docefrez, Taxotere) and paclitaxel (Taxol); Thalidomide (Synovir, Thalomid); and Vinca alkaloids, including vincristine (Vincasar), vinorelbine (Navelbine), and vinblastine (Velban). Treatment of chemotherapy-induced peripheral neuropathy may involve discontinuation or lowering the dose of the anti-cancer drug. Currently, there is no good evidence that any medications, vitamins, or supplements can help you avoid neuropathy.

There are three types of peripheral nerves that can become damaged, causing a wide range of symptoms:

Sensory nerves: Peripheral neuropathy usually affects the sense of touch and feeling in the nerves in the hands and feet. Most individuals feel tingling, burning, pinching, sharp stabs, a buzzing "electrical" sensation, or numbness. It usually starts in the toes and fingers and can continue along the hands and feet toward the body's center. A feeling of wearing tight gloves or stockings is common. An uncomfortable sensation in the hands or feet that may be worse when you touch something is common. Additionally, objects on the feet, such as a shoe or bedcovers, may cause pain. The loss of sensation, may make it difficult to feel hot and cold temperatures or perceive an injury. Another symptom is loss of position sense, which is knowing where one's feet and hands are in space. This may make walking or picking up objects hard, especially if in a dark room or when working with small objects.

Motor nerves: These nerves send information between the brain and muscles. Damage to these nerves can cause difficulty in walking and moving around, and the legs and arms may feel heavy or weak, causing balance and coordination problems. Using the hands and arms may become hard, making everyday tasks, such as brushing teeth more difficult. In addition, muscle cramps and weakening of muscle strength in the hands and feet can occur.

Autonomic nerves: These nerves control involuntary body functions, such as blood pressure and bowel and bladder function. Symptoms include an inability to sweat normally; gastrointestinal issues, such as diarrhea and constipation; dizziness or lightheadedness; trouble swallowing; and sexual dysfunction.

For some individuals, chemotherapy-induced peripheral neuropathy is just a little bothersome and they learn to deal with it. In others, however, it can be so severe that it can lead to stopping chemotherapy or reducing the dosages of the chemotherapeutic agents. Patients experiencing any of these symptoms are encouraged to talk with their physicians or other members of their health care team so that they can get help managing these symptoms.

Persistent neuropathic pain can become a long term problem. **Management** includes relieving the side effects (also called symptom management), and providing palliative care (supportive care). Treatment depends on the cause and the related symptoms. Many individuals recover fully from the condition over time, in a few months or a few years. Sometimes, the disorder may be more difficult to treat and may require long-term management.

There are a number of methods available that may provide some relief:

Medications: Although medications cannot reverse neuropathy, they may relieve the pain. However, they do not relieve the numbness. The most common medications to treat neuropathic pain are anticonvulsants and antidepressants. Over-the-counter pain medications may be recommended for mild pain. Prescription nonsteroidal anti-inflammatory drugs or very strong analgesics may be prescribed for severe pain. Topical treatments, such as lidocaine patches and creams, may also help. However, the medications used to manage neuropathy are related to the specific clinical situation and the cause of the neuropathy.

Nutrition: Eating a diet rich in B vitamins (including B1 and B12), folic acid, and antioxidants may help manage neuropathy. Eating a balanced diet and avoiding excessive alcohol ingestion is recommended.

Physical and/or occupational therapy: Physical and/or occupational therapy can keep muscles strong and improve coordination and balance. Therapists can often recommend assistive devices that can be helpful in completing one's daily activities. Regular exercise may also help reduce pain.

Complementary medicine: Massage, acupuncture, and relaxation techniques may help decrease pain and reduce mental stress.

In severe painful conditions patients may be referred to a **pain management clinic** for a multidisciplinary approach to pain management. Patients who have severe balance problems often benefit from balance (vestibular) rehabilitation.

Home safety can be very important. Enclosed are tips that may help avoid injury in the home for those with sensory or motor difficulties:

- Keeping all rooms, hallways, and stairways well lit
- Installing handrails on both sides of stairways
- Removing small area rugs and any other clutter that could cause one to trip or slip
- Installing grab bars in the shower or hand-grips in the tub, and laying down skid-free mats
- Using a thermometer to check that any water used is below 110^0 F, or setting the water heater accordingly
- Cleaning up any spilled water or liquids immediately
- Using non-breakable dishes
- Using potholders while cooking and rubber gloves when washing dishes
- If driving, making sure that one can fully feel the gas and brake pedals and the steering wheel and that one can quickly move their foot from the gas pedal to the brake pedal
- If prescribed, using a cane or walker when moving from one room to the other

Attention, thinking, and memory problems (cognitive problems)

Many patients who received chemotherapy experience attention, thinking, or short-term memory problems (cognitive problems). Other causes for these issues are pain and other medications, emotional state, and other medical problems.

Read about this at the **Attention, thinking, and memory problems (cognitive problems)** section in **Chapter 3 (page 52)**.

Tiredness (fatigue)

Chemotherapy affects different individuals in different ways. Some people are able to lead a normal life during their treatment, while others may find they become very weak and tired (fatigue) and have to take things more slowly. Any chemotherapy drug may cause fatigue. It can last for a few days or persists through and beyond completion of treatment. Drugs such as vincristine, vinblastine, and cisplatin often cause fatigue.

Read more in the Tiredness (fatigue) section in **Chapter 3 (page 51)**.

More information about the side effects of chemotherapy can be found at the National Cancer Institute (https://www.cancer.gov/publications/patient-education/chemo-side-effects) and Healthline (http://www.healthline.com/health/cancer/effects-on-body) Web sites.

Chapter 5:

Lymphedema, neck swelling, pain and numbness after radiation and surgery for head and neck cancer

Lymphedema

The lymph vessels drain fluid from tissues throughout the body and allow immune cells to travel throughout the body. Lymphedema is a localized lymphatic fluid retention and tissue swelling caused by a compromised lymphatic system.

Lymphedema, a common complication of radiation and surgery for head and neck cancer, is characterized by abnormal accumulation of protein-rich fluid in the space between cells which causes chronic inflammation and reactive fibrosis of the affected tissues.

Radiation creates scarring which interferes with the function of the lymphatics. The cervical lymph nodes are generally removed when the cancer is excised. When the surgeons remove these glands they also take away the drainage system for the lymphatics and cut some of the sensory nerves. Unfortunately, most of the severed lymphatics and nerves are permanently cut. Consequently, it takes longer to drain the area, resulting in swelling. Like flooding after a heavy rain when the drainage system is broken, the surgery creates a backup of lymphatic fluid that cannot drain adequately, as well as numbness of the areas supplied by the severed nerves (usually in the neck, chin, and behind the ears). As a result, some of the lymphatic fluid cannot re-enter the systemic circulation and accumulates in the tissues.

Humid weather and high altitude can aggravate lymphedema. High humidity makes it difficult to perspire and more fluid may accumulates within the body which can increase lymphedema. Also because barometric pressure is reduced at high altitudes, this can lead to the exacerbation of the condition.

There are two types of lymphedema that can develop in patients with head and neck cancer: an **external** visible swelling of the skin or soft tissue and an **internal** swelling of the mucosa of the pharynx and larynx. Lymphedema generally starts slowly and is progressive, rarely painful, causes discomfort in the form of a sensation of heaviness and achiness, and may lead to skin changes.

Lymphedema has several stages:

Stage 0: Latency stage – No visible/palpable edema

Stage 1: Accumulation of protein-rich edema, presence of pitting edema that can be reduced with elevation

Stage 2: Progressive pitting, proliferation of connective tissue (fibrosis)

Stage 3: No pitting, presence of fibrosis, sclerosis, and skin changes

Lymphedema of the head and neck can cause several functional impairments. These include:

- Difficulty in breathing
- Impairment in vision
- Motor limitations (reduced neck motion, jaw tightness or trismus, and chest tightness)
- Sensory limitations
- Speech, voice, and swallowing problems (inability to use an electrolarynx, difficulty in articulation, drooling, and loss of food from mouth)
- Emotional issues (depression, frustration, and embarrassment)

Fortunately over time the lymphatics find newer way of drainage and the swelling generally goes down. Specialists in reducing edema (usually physical therapists) can assist the patient to enhance the drainage and shortening the time for the swelling to decrease. This treatment can also prevent the area from becoming permanently swollen and from developing fibrosis.

Neck tightness and swelling due to lymphedema generally improve over time. Sleeping with the upper body in an elevated position can use gravity to speed the process of lymph fluid drainage.

Treatment of lymphedema includes:

- Manual lymph drainage (Face and neck, deep lymphatics, trunk, intra oral)
- Compressive bandages and garments
- Remedial exercises
- Skin care
- Elastic therapeutic tape (Kinesiotape)
- Oncology rehabilitation

Diuretics, surgical removal (debulking), liposuction, compression pumps, and elevation of the head alone are ineffective treatments. A small clinical trial found that acupuncture and moxibustion (a traditional Chinese medicine therapy using moxa made from dried mugwort) was safe for people with lymphedema, especially when the needles are not put in the area of lymphedema.

A lymphedema treatment specialist can perform and teach manual lymph drainage that can help in reducing edema. Manual lymphatic drainage is a massage-like technique that is performed by specially trained physical therapists. It evolves gentle skin massage to drain edema fluid from the body's periphery into the blood stream towards the heart in an effort to enhance filling of the cutaneous lymph vessels, dilation and contractility of the lymphatic vessels, and recruit unused pathways for lymph flow. Movement and exercise are also important in aiding lymphatic drainage.

A head and neck lymphedema therapist can select **non-elastic bandages** or **compression garments** that are worn at home. These place gentle pressure on the affected areas to help move the lymph fluid and prevent it from refilling and swelling. Application of bandages should be done as directed by a specialist. There are several options, depending on the location of the lymphedema to improve comfort and avoid complications from pressure on the neck.

There are also specific exercises that can reduce the neck tightness and increase the range of neck motion. One needs to perform these exercises throughout life to maintain good neck mobility. This is especially true if the stiffness is due to radiation. Receiving treatment by experienced physical therapies who can also break down the fibrosis is very helpful. The earlier the intervention the better.

A new treatment modality that reduces lymphedema, fibrosis, and neck muscle stiffness using external laser is also available. This method uses a low energy laser beam administered by an experienced physical therapist. The laser beam penetrates into the tissues where it is absorbed by cells and changes their metabolic processes. The beam is generated by the LTU-904 Portable Laser Therapeutic Unit. This treatment can reduce the lymphedema in the neck and face and increase the head's range of motion. It is a painless method that is done by placing the laser instrument at several locations over the neck for about 10 seconds' intervals.

There are physical therapy experts in most communities who specialize in treating lymphedema, and reducing swelling and edema. It is advisable that one consults their surgeon if physical therapy is a good therapeutic option for their lymphedema.

The National Lymphedema Network has a web site that can assist in locating a lymphedema specialists in North America. http://www.lymphnet.org/find-treatment

A facial and neck self-massage guide is also available.
https://ahc.aurorahealthcare.org/fywb/x23169.pdf

Skin numbness after surgery

The cervical lymph nodes, or glands, are generally surgically removed when the cancer is excised. When the surgeons remove these glands, they also cut some of the sensory nerves that supply the lower facial and neck skin. This creates numbness in the areas supplied by the severed nerves. Some of the numb areas may regain sensation in the months following the surgery, but other areas may remain permanently numb.

Most individuals become accustomed to the numbness and are able to prevent damage to the skin from sharp objects, heat or frost. Men learn not to injure the affected area when shaving by using an electric shaver.

The numb skin should be protected from sun burn by applying sunscreen and/or by shielding it with a garment. Frostbite can be prevented by covering the area with a scarf.

Neck and shoulder pain after surgery and radiation

Persistent difficulty with movements of the shoulder, neck, face, and jaw often result from head and neck surgery. These difficulties are the result of the removal or manipulation of the region's muscles, nerves, and lymphatic and blood vessels during surgery and their exposure to radiation therapy. Often, varying degrees of muscle weakness, scar tissue, and lymphedema (see above) are lifelong complications that can affect a person's neck and shoulder health. Because of the proximity of the lymphatic vessels to nerves that innervate the face, neck, and shoulder, they are frequently removed or damaged during surgery of the head and neck. Excision of the cancer may require manipulation or removal of the facial or spinal accessory nerves. The removal of these nerves impacts the movement of face, neck, and shoulder complex muscles.

The effect is generally temporary after nerve manipulation during surgery, but may be permanent if the nerve has been severed. Nevertheless, regeneration of the nerves may occur within six weeks to several years. Following complete severance of the nerves that innervate neck and shoulder muscles, they become limp and fail to stabilize the scapular joints (between the scapula and thorax and the humeral bone). (Figure 2) The affected joints are, therefore, at risk for further injury. When the scapular stabilizer muscles (middle trapezius and rhomboids) are compromised, (Figure 3) it is difficult to maintain an erect posture that allows for proper shoulder retraction. Without adequate retraction of the shoulder girdle, the glenohumeral joint (between the scapula and the humeral bones) cannot elevate the arm through a full range of 180 degrees. Lifting the arm when the scapula is in a protracted (forward) position creates a bony block from the humeral bone hitting the shoulder blade (acromion process) and does not allow full motion.

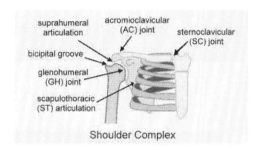

Figure 2: Shoulder complex

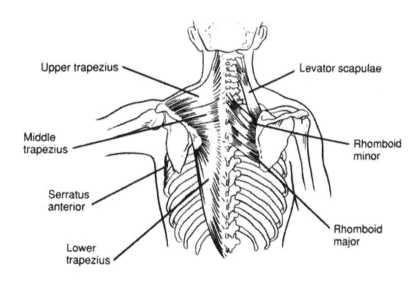

Figure 3: Scapular muscles

Partial dislocation of the shoulder joint (glenohumeral subluxation) can take place because of the lack of muscle stabilization in the shoulder. This creates shoulder instability and an inability to lift the arm through its full range of motion at the shoulder. Further damage to the shoulder joint and rotator cuff can occur with repetitive attempts to use the arm when it is weak. Reduced stability of the joints also creates a structural strain on the neurovascular bundle of the shoulder and surrounding muscles, producing myofascial pain syndrome (chronic dull radiating pain from neck to hand) through the neck, shoulder, and arm. The "leaning forward" posture that gradually develops lengthens the upper back muscles and fascia and shortens the muscles in the chest and neck region. This out of balance posture generates increased strain on the upper back, neck, and shoulder joints.

Radiation therapy further aggravates the situation because of the formation of scar tissue on top of existing scars from the surgical process and complicates one's ability to stretch tight areas. Tissues contractures can also develop in the chest and neck. Scar formation through fibrin formation constitutes the body's healing mechanism following injury and trauma, such as surgery or radiation. The post-surgery process of laying down scar tissue is carried out for about a year. However, since radiation permanently damages DNA and normal cellular processes, scarring typically continues for the rest of the person's life. The fibrin is formed inside and outside the blood vessels, bones, tendons, ligaments and nerves in the affected areas. The resultant condition is called radiation fibrosis syndrome (RFS) and can occur within several weeks or months following radiation. The intensity of the fibrosis depends on the area, the amount and the duration of the radiation. Other factors, such as age and medical comorbidities, also contribute to the amount of RFS created.

Rehabilitation medicine physicians with extensive training in neuromuscular and musculoskeletal medicine, as well as in the principles of functional restoration, are uniquely positioned to improve the quality of life for cancer survivors with radiation fibrosis syndrome. Many factors contribute to neck and shoulder pain after surgery in the neck region. Education and active participation in the management process after surgery of the head and neck are important to minimizing the resulting discomfort. One should contact a physical and/or occupational therapist to help gather all the tools needed to manage chronic changes.

Chapter 6:

Methods of speaking after laryngectomy

Although total laryngectomy removes the entire larynx (vocal cords/voice box), most laryngectomees can acquire a new way of speaking. About 85-90% of laryngectomees learn to speak using one of the three main methods of speaking described below. About 10% do not communicate by speaking but can use computer-based or other methods to communicate.

Individuals normally speak by exhaling air from their lung to vibrate their vocal cords. These vibration sounds are modified in the mouth, by the tongue, lips, and teeth to generate the sounds that create speech. Although the vocal cords that are the source of the vibrating sounds are removed during total laryngectomy, other forms of speech can be created by using a new pathway for air and a different airway part to vibrate. Another method is to generate vibration by an artificial source placed on the outside of the throat or mouth and then using the mouth parts to form speech.

The method(s) used to speak again depend on the type of surgery. Some people may be limited to a single method, while others may have several choices. Each method has unique characteristics, advantages and disadvantages. The goal of attaining a new way to speak is to meet the communication needs of each laryngectomee.

Patient education about the available speech choice after laryngectomy is essential both before and after surgery. Speech and language pathologists (SLPs) can assist and guide laryngectomees in the proper use of the methods and/or devices they use to obtain the most understandable speech. Speech improves considerably between six months and one year after total laryngectomy. Active voice rehabilitation is associated with attaining better functional speech.

The three main methods of speaking after laryngectomy are:

Tracheoesophageal speech

This method provides the most natural sounding voice, is loud, requires a puncture connecting the trachea and esophagus and a prosthesis that is inserted into it.

The method requires placing the silicone voice prosthesis that is inserted into a puncture (called tracheoesophageal puncture or TEP) created by the surgeon. (**Figure 4**) The hole is made at the back of the trachea (the windpipe) and goes into the esophagus (food tube). The hole between the trachea and esophagus can be done at the same time as the laryngectomy surgery (a primary puncture), or after healing from the surgery has occurred (a secondary puncture). A small tube called a voice prosthesis, is inserted in this hole and prevents the puncture from closing. It has a one-way valve at the end on the esophagus side which allows air to go into the esophagus but prevents swallowed liquids from coming through the prosthesis and reaching the trachea and lungs.

Speaking is possible by diverting the exhaled air through the prosthesis into the esophagus by temporarily occluding the stoma. This can be done by sealing it with a finger or by pressing on a special Heat and Moisture Exchange (HME) filter that is worn over the stoma. An HME partially restores the lost nasal functions. Some use a "hands free" HME (automatic speaking valve) that is activated by speaking.

After occlusion of the stoma exhaled lung air moves through the prosthesis into the esophagus causing the walls and top of the esophagus to vibrate. These vibrations are used by the mouth (tongue, lips, teeth, etc.) to create the sounds of speech.

There are two different basic types of voice prosthesis: the patient-changed type, designed to be changed by the laryngectomee or by another person, and the indwelling type, designed to be changed by a medical professional (an otolaryngologist or SLP).

The HME or automatic speaking valve can be attached in front of the tracheostoma in different ways: by means of an adhesive housing that is taped or glued to the skin, or by means of a laryngectomy tube or stoma button that is placed inside the stoma.

The voice prosthesis need to be periodically replaced (this is covered by some medical insurances). This method requires obtaining supplies, daily up keeping and cleaning, dealing with failure of the TEP mostly due to leakage (see **Chapter 10, pages 150-156**) , and the prosthesis may need adjustments and individual fitting.

Patients who use TEP have the best results in speech intelligibility 6 months and one year after total laryngectomy. The larger the inner diameter of the prosthesis, the stronger is the voice and the easier it is to speak.

Speech can be made clearer and easier by:

- Speaking slowly
- Speaking only 4-5 words between each air exhalation
- Using diaphragmatic breathing (see below)
- Over articulating the words
- Speaking by using low air pressure

Laryngectomees often try to compensate for their low volume by increasing the exhalation air pressure. This is tiring and can lead to air leak around the HME's base plate.

Individuals who suffer from chronic obstructive pulmonary disease (COPD) may have difficulties using tracheoesophageal speech and may find it impossible to use hands free HME.

Speech can also be improved by enhancing air flow. This can be achieved by relaxing the throat muscles, breathing deep breathes (preferably using diaphragmatic breathing) (see below), and lubricating the airways by drinking. Drinking water also relaxes the throat muscles.

It is important to make sure that the adhesive housing is sealed and not leaking air (see **Heat moisture exchanger filter care** in **Chapter 9, page 136**).

Tracheoesophageal Voice Prosthesis

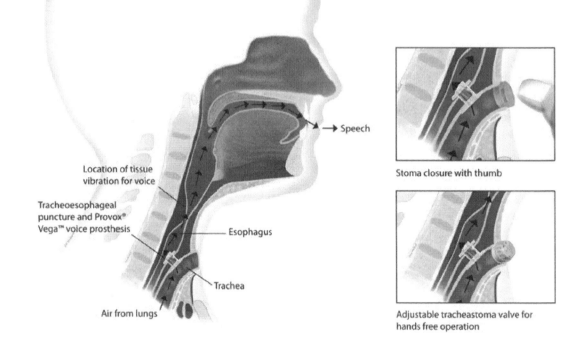

Figure 4: Tracheoesophageal speech

Esophageal speech

Esophageal speech is produced by insufflating the esophagus with air and then allowing this air to be released through the upper esophageal sphincter where vibration creates sound. (**Figure 5**) This method does not require any instrumentation.

In contrast to tracheoesophageal speech, which occurs when pulmonary air is shunted through a prosthesis, esophageal speech relies on active air insufflation from the mouth. Air can enter the esophagus only when there is higher pressure above the upper esophageal sphincter than below.

Thus, air insufflation occurs either when patients produce high intra-oral pressure or when they create low pressure at the level of the upper esophageal sphincter by relaxing the cricopharyngeus muscle.

Esophageal speech training includes training in strategies to accomplish air insufflation as well as treatment of distracting secondary behaviors. Positive pressure injection methods rely on using the articulators to force high-pressure air through the cricopharyngeus while the inhalation method relies on chest expansion and dropping of upper esophageal pressures to pull air into the esophagus.

Of the three major types of speech following laryngectomy, esophageal speech usually takes longest to learn. However, it has several *advantages*, not the least of which includes freedom from dependency on devices and instrumentation, it does not require purchasing any equipment and is hands free. *Disadvantages* include the need for training, slow speaking rate, often lower volume and dependency on the function of the cricoparyngeal muscle and pharyngeal segment. Some SLPs are familiar with esophageal speech and can and assist laryngectomees in learning this method. Self-help books and tapes can also help in learning this method of speech.

Esophageal Speech

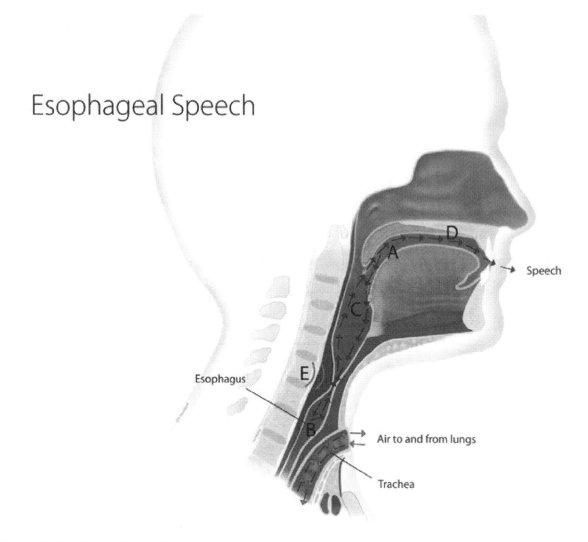

Figure 5: Esophageal speech

Electrolarynx or artificial larynx speech

This method of speaking is quickly and easily learned, produces a strong sound, is powerful, requires a device with batteries, and the use of one hand. It also requires manually dexterity, and the ability to turn the device on before and off after speaking.

The vibrations in this speech method are generated pneumatically by an external battery operated vibrator (called electrolarynx or artificial-larynx) which is usually placed on the cheek or under the chin. (**Figure 6**)

It makes a buzzing vibration that reaches the throat and mouth of the user. The person then modifies the sound using his/her mouth to articulate the speech sounds.

There are three methods to deliver the vibration sounds created by an artificial larynx into the throat and mouth (intra orally). One is directly into the mouth by a straw-like tube (i.e., the Cooper Rands electrolarynx) and the other through the skin of the neck or face. In the last method, which produces the best results the electrolarynx (EL) is held against the face or neck. A denture type artificial larynx is also available. However, it is rarely used and has limited success in phonation.

ELs are often used by laryngectomees shortly after their laryngectomy while they are still hospitalized. Because of the neck swelling and post-surgical stitches the intra oral route of delivery of vibration is preferred at that time. The best placement of the intra oral straw (adaptor) need to be individually explored. It generally works best to place the straw far enough in the mouth to allow the sound to resonate. If it is placed too far forward, the sound may not be audible. The straw should not be placed in the side of mouth and its head should not be placed under the tongue or check. Many laryngectomees can learn other methods of speaking later. However, they can still use an EL on as their main speaking methods or as a back-up in case they encounter problems with their other speaking methods (i.e., a blown baseplate seal, excess mucous, a plugged or blocked TEP).

Even though using an EL is not hard, practicing and acquiring the correct technique can improve communication and ensure one is understood. It is also important the device be in adequate working order. There are several adjustments that can be made to the device to assist in achieving the best quality speech possible. The SLP can adjust and teach the laryngectomee how to troubleshoot this device as needed to ensure production of understandable speech.

Although it may be frustrating to use at first, with proper training and practice, most people can become very effective EL speakers in a very short period of time. If possible, it is a good idea to hold and operate the EL in one's non-dominant hand since it frees up the other hand.

Tips that can assist in improving speech include:

- *"Head" Placement*: The head of the EL has to be placed in full contact with the skin surface of the neck. Even beard whiskers can interfere with proper contact and voice production.

- *Contact pressure:* For best vocalization results the contact pressure of the "head" should be adequate. This is achieved by trial and error. Too little pressure enhances external vibration noises, while too much pressure decreases the sound.

- *Proper Positioning:* For every laryngectomee there are areas of higher or lower resonance in the throat. This is determined mostly by the density or thickness of the neck tissues at that location. The most ideal placement is generally in a location where the neck tissues are thinner and softer, at a level where there is space in the throat to resonate. In general, the more dense or "tough" the neck tissues are, the harder it will be to produce a good tone.

- *The "Sweet Spot":* There is generally an individual "sweet spot" (perfect position) where the EL produces the best resonant tone. This can be found by placing the EL at various positions around the neck, under the chin and even on the cheek. The sweet spot can change over time as healing progresses.

- Improving articulation: The typical EL user needs to change their speech pattern somewhat in order to be well understood. It is helpful to articulate more precisely and over articulate; speaking only 4-5 words in each air exhalation; speak slowly, clearly and concisely; and remembering to do that with an open mouth. Taking time to articulate each sound is important.

- Turning the device on and off at appropriate times can significantly impact how well others understand the speech. The device should be turned on at the same time as one starts speaking and turned off at the end of a short phrase or at a natural pause to reduce the unnecessary mechanical buzz. It is important to avoiding turning the device on for each individual word or keep it on for an entire conversation without a break. Short phrases are the easiest for conversational partners to understand.

- Avoiding forced air exhalation while speaking to reduce audible rushes of air ("stoma blast")

Electrolarynx mechanism of Speech

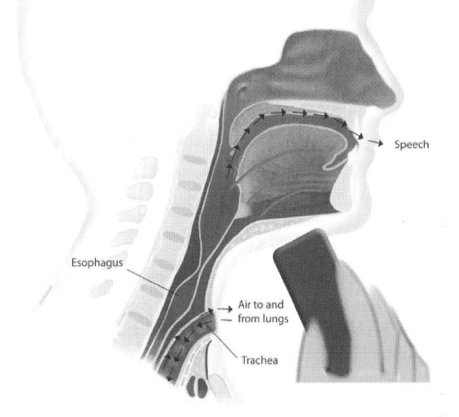

Figure 6: Electrolarynx or artificial larynx speech

Other methods of speech and communication

A **pneumatic artificial larynx** (also called Tokyo Artificial Larynx) is also available to generate speech. This method uses lung air to vibrate a reed or rubber material that produces a sound. The device's cup is placed over the stoma and its tube is inserted in the mouth. (**Picture 1**) The sound generated is injected into the mouth through the tube. It does not use any batteries and is relatively inexpensive.

Those who are unable to use any of the above methods can use speech generated devices such as computer generated speech using either a standard laptop computer, or a single purpose speech aid. (See below) The user types what he/she wants to say onto a keyboard, and the computer speaks out loud what has been typed. Smart phones and some cell phones can also operate in this manner.

Sending written messages and texting through mobile phones (smart phones, or cell phones) and computers can help laryngectommees communicate in noisy places or when they have other communication difficulties.

Other methods of communication can use the assistance of a companion who knows and understands the laryngectomee; writing messages with a pencil or pen, or on an erase board; using sign language, gestures or facial expressions; and by predetermined clicks.

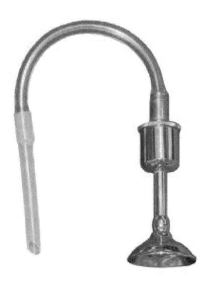

Picture 1: Pneumatic artificial larynx

Speech generating devices

Speech-generating devices produce a pre-recorded or electronic message in response to pressing a button or icon. There are many devices available and include smartphones, laptops, androids and iPhones. There are programs that convert a written language into speech.

Many individuals with communication impairments including laryngectomees are using their personal electronic devices (i.e., laptop, smartphone, etc.) generate speech. Any computer can be used as speech generating device (SGD) by enabling its user to input a message that the computer then speak aloud.

Laryngectomees can use SGDs for communication in one or more of the following ways:

- For communication after surgery until they regain speech through use of a voice prosthesis, EL or esophageal speech.
- As the main communication method for those who are unable to regain speech because of extensive surgery or other reasons.
- As a secondary communication method to clarify their spoken messages when they are not easily understood or where they anticipate difficulty being understood (i.e., noisy environment, using the telephone, etc.)
- As a backup method for occasional use when there is difficulty with their speech method (e.g., their electrolarynx is broken).

Many devices can be used as an SGD after installing appropriate programs or applications.

There are two types of SGDs:

- *Integrated Devices:* Devices such as laptop computers, desktop computers, smartphones or tablets can function as an SGD after installation of a program or application.

- *Dedicated Devices:* These SGDs are designed for communication. They are regarded as medical equipment and require a physician's prescription. Their design typically includes an adequate speaker, various voice options, and multi-functional communication software.

Evaluation by a SLP is advisable when considering obtaining an SGD. The SLP can assist in the selection and evaluation process and arrange for trials of different devices.

Selection of the most appropriate SGD requires considering how they are to be used:

- Is it to be used in or outside home, at work, on the telephone, or all of these?
- Will it be the main method used in conjunction with one's speech?
- Determining the size and weight of an SGD is based on one's vision and ability to carry it.
- Selecting the number of available features in an SGD depends on one's comfort using this technology.

Some available features make the use of an SGD easier through auto prediction and auto correction.

SGD can assist in communication over the phone: A speakerphone is placed near the SGD and the message can be typed into the SGD which speaks it aloud. The speakerphone picks up the computerized voice and sends it out. It is helpful to begin conversations by telling the other person that one is using a computer to talk, so that the listener will know it is a person on the other end and not an automated call.

The SGD's volume can be increased as needed with the addition of a small speaker that plugs into the device.

Some speech generating software and applications are available at no cost and others are sold at different prices. Expensive ones offer better voice quality and more features (e.g., the ability to store frequently used messages, word prediction, ability to vary the speech settings, etc.). Many of the more expensive programs offer either a free trial period or the ability to download a rudimentary version of the application at no cost. This allows one to try the basic features of the software and see if it fits one's needs before making the purchase.

Medicare and private insurances generally cover a portion of the cost of dedicated devices, and may cover the purchase of speech generating software programs. However, they do not provide funding to purchase a computer to be used as an SGD. Purchasing an SGD through Medicare or insurance, requires an evaluated by an SLP who will document one's need for the device. The state of Oregon provides an SGD through their telephone assistance program.

Speaking on the phone

Speaking over the phone is often difficult for laryngectomees. Their voice is sometimes hard to understand and some individuals may even hang up the phone when they hear them.

It is best to inform the other party about the speaking difficulties of the laryngectomee by first asking them "can you hear me?" This may enable the larynngectomee to inform and explain to their party about their speaking difficulties.

It is important to articulate clearly when speaking over the phone. One should speak slowly and even "over articulate" words. Those who converse with a laryngectomee can read their lips during face-to-face conversation. This is of course not possible over the phone. However, speaking through a video call (such as with Skype) allows for lip reading. One can practice phone conversation (without lip reading) by speaking to someone in person while not facing them.

Tips that can help electrolarynx (EL) users include:

- Place the phone's microphone right at the lips, or slightly above them. Placing the microphone close to the EL introduces some of the buzzing sounds which would make it more difficult to be understood.
- Articulate your words very carefully.
- Turn the EL volume down. With the phone's microphone close to the mouth, the EL sounds can be very low. Louder EL sounds might masks one's articulation and make it difficult to be understood.

There are phones available that can amplify the outgoing voice, making it easier for the laryngectomee to be heard and understood.

There is a nationwide phone service that allows a person whose speech may be difficult to understand to communicate over the telephone with the help of a specially trained communications assistant. No special telephone is needed for this calling option. The three digit number 711 can be used as a shortcut to access Telecommunications Relay Services (TRS) anywhere in the U.S. TRS facilitates telephone conversations by one or more people who have speech and hearing disabilities. All telecommunications carriers in the U.S., including wire-line, wireless and pay phone providers must provide 711 service.

Sending written messages (texting) through mobile phones (smart phones, or cell phones) can help laryngectommees communicate in noisy places or when they have other communication difficulties.

Other communication methods include teletypewriter devices (TTY), telecommunication device for the deaf (TDD), and using a telephone modem and display between devices, and using relay operators.

Diaphragmatic breathing and speech

Diaphragmatic breathing (also called abdominal breathing) is the act of breathing slowly and deeply by using the diaphragm muscle rather than by using one's rib cage muscles. When breathing using the diaphragm, the abdomen, rather than the chest expands. This method of breathing allows for greater utilization of the lung capacity to obtain oxygen, dispose of bicarbonate gasses, and increases air flow.

Neck breathers are often shallow breathers who use a relatively smaller portion of their lung capacity. Becoming accustomed to inhaling by using the diaphragm can increase one's stamina and also improve esophageal and tracheoesophageal speech by enhancing the ability to speak and increasing the voice volume.

Diaphragmatic breathing is also relaxing and can be used to decrease general anxiety, tension, and perception of pain.

This breathing method can be taught by a speech and language pathologist.

Using a voice amplifier

One of the problems encountered when using tracheoesophageal or esophageal speech is the weakness of the volume. Using a waistband voice amplifier enables one to speak with less effort and can allow one to be heard even in noisy places. It also prevents breakage of the stoma's housing seal because the laryngectomee who uses tracheoesophageal speech does not need to generate a strong expiratory air pressure to exhale air though the voice prosthesis.

Using a microphone with a foam windscreen cover makes the voice clearer and reduces unwanted background noises created by the lips. Holding the microphone close to the lips, having the windscreen touching the lower lip is best. Ideally it should never be more than 1/4 inch away.

Chapter 7:

Mucus and respiratory care, humidifiers, blowing the nose and coping with cold or warm weather after laryngectomy

---

Mucus production is the body's way of protecting and maintaining the health of the trachea (windpipe) and lungs. It serves to lubricate these airways and keep them moist. Following laryngectomy, the trachea opens at the stoma and a laryngectomee can no longer cough up mucus and then swallow it, or blow the nose. It is still very important to cough and clear one's mucus; however, this must be done through the stoma.

Immediately after surgery, the patient's tracheal secretions increases and may be difficult to clear. While hospitalized tracheal suctioning is done by the hospital staff, and the patient and their caregivers should learn how to perform suctioning using sterile techniques prior to discharge. For the first 3-4 months many laryngectomees require tracheal suctioning as an adjunct to coughing to clear their airways. Over time mucous production slowly decreases. This is enhanced by wearing a Heat and Moisture Exchanger (HME). Also, over time, most patients are able to produce adequate coughing strength to expel secretions without the need for a suction device.

Coughing up mucus through the stoma is the only way by which laryngectomees can keep their trachea and lungs clear of dust, dirt, micro-organisms (bacteria, viruses and fungi), and other contaminants that may get into their airways. It is therefore important to protect the airways from inhalation of these by covering the stoma preferably by a stoma cover or HME filter. Whenever an urge to cough or sneeze emerges laryngectomees must quickly remove their stoma cover or HME and use a tissue or handkerchief to cover their stoma to catch the mucus.

The best mucus consistency is clear, or almost clear, and watery. Such consistency, however, is not easy to maintain because of changes in the environment and weather. Steps can be routinely taken to maintain a healthy mucus production as shown below.

Humidity and humidifiers

Humidity is the amount of water in the air. The amount of humidity can vary depending on the season of the year, weather and the location. Usually, humidity levels are elevated in the summer months and lower during winter. The ideal, home humidity for neck breathers should be between 40-50 %. Humidity that's too low or too high can cause medical problems.

Low humidity can cause dry skin, irritate ones nasal passages and throat, and make one's eyes itchy.

High humidity can make the home feel stuffy and can cause condensation of water on walls, floors and other surfaces that enhances the growth of molds, bacteria, and dust mites. These allergens can cause respiratory problems and trigger allergy and asthma flare-ups.

The best way to test humidity levels in one's house is by using a hygrometer. The hygrometer appears like a thermometer, and measures the amount of moisture in the air. It is available at hardware and department stores. When purchasing a humidifier, it is wise to get one with a built-in hygrometer (humidistat) that can maintain humidity within the healthy range.

Humidifiers emit water vapor or steam that increase moisture levels in the air (humidity).

There are several types of humidifiers:

- **Central humidifiers** are constructed within the home as part of the heating and air conditioning systems and are built to humidify the entire house.
- **Ultrasonic humidifiers** generate a cool mist through ultrasonic vibration.
- **Impeller humidifiers** create a cool mist by a rotating disk.
- **Evaporators** use a fan that blows air through a wet wick, filter or belt.
- **Steam vaporizers** use electricity to generate steam that cools down before exciting the machine. These kind of humidifier should be avoided around children because of potential burn injury.

- **Nebulizer bottle** is used to turn saline into smaller particles to be delivered to the stoma or breathing tube.

Keeping the humidifier clean

Humidifiers generally come with instructions by the manufacturer how to keep them clean. Unplugging the humidifier before changing water or cleaning it is mandatory.

Enclosed are tips how to keep portable humidifiers free of harmful mold, fungi and bacteria:

Using only distilled or demineralized water. Tap water contains minerals that can deposit inside the humidifier and enhance bacterial growth. When these minerals are released into the air, they can be inhaled into the trachea and lungs and frequently appear as white dust on the furniture. Distilled or demineralized water contain a much lower amount of minerals compared with tap water. Many manufacturers recommend the use of demineralization cartridges or filters.

Changing humidifier water frequently. Film or deposits develop inside humidifiers if their water is not changed on a regular basis. Empting the tanks, drying the inside surfaces and refilling the humidifier with clean water on a daily basis is recommended, especially when using cool mist or ultrasonic humidifiers.

Cleaning humidifiers every 3 days. Mineral deposits or film in the tank or other parts of the humidifier should be removed preferably by using a 3 % hydrogen peroxide solution. Chlorine bleach or other disinfectants are recommended by some manufacturers. The tank should be rinsed after cleaning to remove harmful chemicals that can become airborne and inhaled.

Changing humidifier filters on a regular basis. Filters in humidifiers, and in the central air conditioning and heating system, should be changed according to the manufacturer recommend- or whenever they become dirty.

Keeping the area around humidifiers dry. The humidifier should be turned down whenever the area or objects around them become damp or wet.

Proper preparation of humidifiers for storage. The humidifier should be drained and cleaned prior to storage and whenever they are taken out of storage for use. All used cartridges, cassettes or filters should be discarded.

Following instructions for central humidifiers. Humidifier built into the central heating and cooling system should be maintained according to their manufacturer's instruction manual.

Replacing old humidifiers. With the passage of time, deposits can build up in humidifiers that are difficult or impossible to remove and promote the growth of bacteria and fungi. It is best to replace them.

Features of Warm and Cool Mist Humidifiers

Humidifiers help maintain a healthy humidity level in moisture-deprived locations. Humidifiers can add moisture using either warm or cool mist technologies. Both types have their strengths and weaknesses.

Both humidifier types help avoid the unwanted effects of dry air, which can include irritation of the laryngectomee's upper airways that may lead to respiratory ailments.

Cool Mist Humidifiers: Cool mist humidifiers disperse a comfortable stream of room-temperature mist. These humidifiers are available in evaporative or ultrasonic technologies. Cool mist evaporative humidifiers use an internal wick filter to absorb water while a fan blows the air through the filter. This process causes the water to evaporate throughout the room as an ultra-fine, invisible mist. Cool mist ultrasonic humidifiers use ultrasonic vibration technology to create a micro-fine cool mist that is quietly released throughout the environment.

Because the water is not heated before it is dispersed, these humidifiers typically use less electricity. The use of cool mist humidifiers avoids getting burns because of hot water accidents.

One drawback to cool mist evaporative humidifiers, however, is noise. Since these devices use fans to blanket the room with moisture, they can be slightly noisier than other humidifier types. Additionally, the cool mist can cause the air to feel slightly chillier than usual.

Warm Mist Humidifiers: Warm mist humidifiers use an internal heating element that boils water before releasing it into the environment as a soothing invisible mist. These humidifiers are often considered healthier since the boiling process kills waterborne bacteria and mold, which prevents them from entering the airways. The absence of an internal fan makes warm mist humidifiers exceptionally quiet to operate. Warm mist humidifiers are also available in ultrasonic models.

Warm mist humidifiers are not as well-suited for large areas as cool mist models. Instead, these humidifiers work best in smaller areas like bedrooms and offices. In addition, warm mist humidifiers are slightly more expensive to operate and a little more difficult to clean since mineral deposits are often left behind during the boiling process. However, many people have found these humidifiers to be more comfortable for use during cold winter months.

Mucus production and increasing air humidity

Prior to becoming a laryngectomee, the inhaled air is warmed to body temperature, humidified and cleansed of organisms and dust particles by the filtration capacity of the upper part of the respiratory system. Since these functions do not occur following laryngectomy, it is important to restore the lost functions previously provided by upper part of the respiratory system.

Followed laryngectomy the inhaled air does not get humidified and filtered by passing through the nose and mouth; accordingly, tracheal dryness, irritation and overproduction of mucus develops. Fortunately, the trachea becomes more tolerant to dry air over time. However, when the humidity level is too low the trachea can dry out, crack, and produce some bleeding. If the bleeding is significant or does not respond to an increase in humidity, a physician should be consulted. And if the amount or color of the mucus is concerning, one should contact a physician.

Tracheal dryness, irritation and overproduction of mucus can lead to the development of mucus plugs. These plugs can cause airway obstruction that can lead to collapse of sections (atelectasis) of the lungs.

Restoring the humidification of the inhaled air reduces the overproduction of mucus to an adequate level and reduce the risk of mucus plugs. This will decrease the chances for coughing unexpectedly and plugging the HME filter. Those without an HME need to cover their stoma with a paper towel or even their hand to collect the coughed mucus. Increasing the home humidity to 40-50% relative humidity (not higher) can help in decreasing mucus production and keeping the stoma and trachea from drying out, cracking and bleeding. In addition to being painful, these cracks can also become pathways for infections.

Saline bullets are commonly used to provide quick moisture to the lower airways. These plastic bullets contain 3-10 cc sterile saline and after their tip is broken their contents is squeezed through the stoma into the trachea. The insertion of saline induces immediate coughing that facilitates the clearing of secretions. The contents of the bullets is introduced by several insertions. It is generally useful to use saline bullets as needed several times a day or as directed by one's physician.

Steps to achieve better humidification and healthier mucus production include:

- Wearing an HME 24/7 which keeps the tracheal moisture higher and preserves the heat inside the trachea and lungs
- Wetting the soma cover (or bib) to breathe moist air (in those who wear a stoma cover). Although less effective than an HME, dampening the foam filter or stoma cover with clean plain water can also assist in increasing humidification.
- Drinking enough fluid to keep well hydrated

- Inserting 3-5 cc saline (preferably using saline "Bullets") into the stoma at least twice a day (see below how to prepare saline)
- Using a humidifier in the house to achieve about 40-50% humidity and getting a hygrometer to monitor the humidity. This is important both in the summer when air conditioning is used, and in the winter when heating is used
- Using nebulizing bottle twice daily
- Breathing steam generated by boiling water or a hot shower

A digital humidity gauge (called a hygrometer) can assist in controlling the humidity levels. Over time, as the airways adjusts, the need to always use a humidifier may decrease.

Preparing saline solution

Saline solution is a salt solution, which can be prepared using readily available materials. This recipe is for a salt solution that is normal (0.9%), which means it is the same concentration or isotonic to body fluids. Because the salt composition is similar to that of the body, it causes less tissue damage than pure water. Saline solution consists of sodium chloride (table salt) in water. When using the solution to clean a wound or for squirting it into the trachea, it's important to use pure ingredients and maintain sterile conditions.

It is important to use uniodized salt, which does not have iodine added to it, and avoid using rock salt or sea salt, since they have added chemicals. Using distilled water or reverse osmosis purified water is preferred over ordinary tap water.

To prepare the saline one need to mix 1 teaspoon of salt per 2 cups (500 ml fluid) of water. To obtain a sterile solution, the salt is dissolved in boiling water. The solution can be kept sterile by placing a lid over the container so that no microorganisms get into the liquid or air space as the solution cools.

The sterile solution can be dispensed into sterile containers. The containers can be sterilized by boiling them in water for one minute. It's a good idea to label the container with the date and to discard it if the solution is not used within a few days. It's important to avoid contaminating the liquid, so ideally make just as much solution as you need at a time, allow it to cool, and discard leftover liquid. The sterile solution will remain suitable for use for several days in its sealed container, but you should expect some degree of contamination once it is opened.

The saline can be squirted into the stoma using a sterile squirting bulb.

Caring for the airways and neck in cold weather and a high altitude

Winter and high altitude can be rough for laryngectomees. The air at high altitude is thinner containing less oxygen and colder and therefore dryer. Before laryngectomy air is inhaled through the nose where it becomes warm and moist before entering the lungs. After a laryngectomy the air is no longer inhaled through the nose and enters the trachea directly through the stoma. Cold air is dryer than warm air and more irritating to the trachea. This is because cold air contains less humidity and therefore can dry the trachea and cause bleeding. The mucus can also become dry and plug the trachea.

Breathing cold air can also have an irritating effect on the airways causing the smooth muscle that surrounds the airways to contract (bronchospasm). This decreases the size of the airways and makes it hard to get the air in and out of the lungs causing shortness of breath. In very cold weather the moisture in the HME can freeze making it even harder to breathe. When this occurs replacing the HME can bring some relief.

Caring for the airways includes the steps described in **pages 111-112** as well as:

- Avoid exposure to cold, dry or dusty air
- Avoid dust, irritants and allergens
- When exposed to cold air, consider covering the stoma with a jacket (by zipping it all the way) or a loose scarf or bandana and breathing into the space between the jacket and the

body to warm the inhaled air. Another option is to wear a scarf or a thin T-shirt over the face; that cover the nose, mouth, and stoma; like a mask. This will keep the neck and face warm and create a space for the exhaled and inhaled air to warm up and stay humid. It also allows for air filtration and oxygen and bicarbonate exchange with the environment.

- Temporary removal of the HME under a cover (see above) can be helpful allowing greater air exchange
- Replace a frozen HME with a new one
- Keep the airway humid by wearing an HME and inserting saline bullets
- Cough out or suctioning the mucus using a suction machine to clean the airways

Following a laryngectomy which involves neck dissection most individuals develop areas of numbness in their neck, chin and behind the ears. Consequently they cannot sense cold air and can develop frostbite at these sites. It is therefore important to cover these areas with a scarf or garment.

Laryngectomees and hot weather

Hot weather is generally easier on a laryngectomee because of the increased air humidity. However, similar to non-laryngectomees it is important to take precautions and stay well hydrated (preferably by drinking cold drinks), avoid direct sun exposure, wear light lose cloth, cover the head, and stay indoors if the quality of air is poor.

Those at greatest risk of heat-related illnesses are people aged 65 years and older. Exposure to extreme heat has particularly adverse effects on people with chronic illnesses such as respiratory, cardiovascular, and renal diseases, diabetes, obesity, and mental illness. Medications including blood pressure and heart medicine (beta-blockers), water pills (diuretics), antidepressants, antipsychotics and anticonvulsants (seizure medication) and antihistamines (allergy medications) may also affect how the body reacts to heat.

Laryngectomees should keep in touch with friends and family, as they may be their lifeline in case they need assistance. Wearing a heat and moisture exchanger (HME) reduces water loss through the lungs that can contribute to dehydration.

Using suction machine to clear secretions and mucus plugs

A suction machine is often used by new laryngectomee in the hospital and in the immediate period after they are discharged from hospital. During this period forceful coughing is difficult and suctioning is used to clear the mucus. However, it is important to learn to cough out mucus and clear one's secretions without a suction machine. A deep and strong cough is more effective than a suction machine in removing respiratory secretions. However, there may be individuals that require the use of a suction machine for a longer period.

A suction machine can, however, can be used to suction out mucus when one is unable to cough it out and/or to remove a mucus plug. A mucus plug can develop when the mucus become thick and sticky creating a plug that blocks part or, infrequently, even the whole airway.

The plug can cause a sudden and unexplained shortness of breath. A suction machine can be used in these circumstances to remove the plug. It should therefore be readily available to treat such an emergency. Mucus plugs may also be removed by using a saline "bullet" (0.9% sterile salt water in a plastic tube) or by squirting saline solution into the stoma. The saline can loosen the plug that can be coughed out. This condition may become a medical emergency, and if the plug is not successfully removed after several attempts dialing 911 may be lifesaving.

Coughing blood

Blood in the mucus can originate from several sources. The most common is from a scratch just inside the stoma. The scratch can be caused by trauma while cleaning the stoma. The blood generally appears bright red. Another common cause of coughing blood in a laryngectomee is irritation of the trachea because of dryness which is common during the winter.

Possible causes of minimal bleeding include:

- Irritation to the fragile tissue around the stoma
- Insufficient humidity to the airway
- Too frequent, deep or vigorous suctioning
- Suction pressure that is too high (Suction machine pressure for adults 100-120 mm Hg)
- Infection
- Trauma, manipulation of trach
- Foreign object in the airway
- Excessive coughing

It is advisable to maintain a home environment with adequate humidity levels (about 40-50%) to also help minimize drying the trachea. Wearing a heat and moisture exchanger (HME) 24/7 (See HME filter care section) and inserting sterile saline into the stoma can help. (See above in the "Mucus production section")

RT after laryngectomy can cause local inflammation and bloodstained mucus. Bloody sputum can also be a symptom of pneumonia, tuberculosis, lung cancer, or other lung problem. Persistent coughing of blood should be evaluated by medical professionals. This may be urgent if it is associated with difficulties in breathing and/or pain.

Lower respiratory infections (bronchitis, tracheitis, and tracheobronchitis) in laryngectomees

Laryngectomees are directly exposed to airborne respiratory pathogens (i.e., viruses, bacteria) because the air they inhale is no longer filtered by the nasal mucosa. This makes them more susceptible to lower respiratory tract and other infections that access the body through the respiratory tract.

Following laryngectomy the tracheal epithelium also becomes directly exposed to the relatively cold and dry ambient air entering the tracheostoma.

This can causes:

- Drying of the mucus (altered mucus viscosity)
- Reduction of ciliary activity that causes impaired mucociliary clearance
- Tracheal epithelium damage (loss of ciliated cells, goblet cell hyperplasia, and excessive mucus production and metaplasia).

Laryngectomized patients have considerable pulmonary complaints such as frequent coughing and forceful expectoration of sputum. Laryngectomees also run a higher risk of developing severe respiratory infections.

Severe pulmonary infections (tracheobronchitis or pneumonia) in laryngectomees are more frequent in wintertime and the accompanying tracheal crusting often requires antibiotic treatment or even hospitalization.

The stoma allows the inhaled air to bypasses the natural defenses (nasal hair and mucus membranes) of the upper airway that filter out dust and bacteria. The number of bronchitis, tracheobronchitis, and pneumonia episodes as well as mortality due to these infections in non-HME users was found to be 3 times higher than in HME users. Laryngectomees especially those who do not wear an HME or do not cover their stoma are therefore at a higher risk of developing lower respiratory tract infections.

Bronchitis is an inflammation of the lining of the bronchial tubes, which carry air to and from the lungs. People who have bronchitis often cough up thickened mucus, which can be discolored. Acute bronchitis can develop from a cold or other respiratory infection.

Symptoms of bronchitis include:

- Cough
- Production of mucus (sputum), which can be clear, white, yellowish-gray or green in color- rarely, it may be streaked with blood
- Fatigue
- Shortness of breath
- Slight fever and chills
- Chest discomfort
- Mild headache or body aches.

While these symptoms usually improve in about a week, a nagging cough can linger for several weeks.

Treatment of bronchitis in laryngectomees is more challenging.

Managing bronchitis in a laryngectomee requires:

- Keeping the stoma open by manually removing accumulates mucus that can dry out and clog it.
- Keeping the excessive sputum moist by breathing humidified air and inserting saline "bullets" as needed
- Coughing out or suctioning accumulated sputum
- Removing the stoma cover prior to coughing to prevent blocking it with the coughed out sputum
- Use thick paper tissues or handkerchiefs to pick up any coughed mucus. Do not use thin absorbing paper such as toilet paper or tissues, as they can be suctioned into the stoma
- Keeping well hydrated

- Wearing an HME may be difficult during bronchitis as the excessive mucus may prevent it from adhering to the skin around the stoma.
- Elevating one's head and chest while sleeping
- Using medication prescribed by one's physician (such as bronchodilators, fever reducing medications, and expectorants).

Because most cases of bronchitis are caused by viral infections, antibiotics are not effective. However, if one's doctor suspects a bacterial infection, he or she may prescribe an antibiotic.

Tracheitis and tracheobronchitis can be caused by a virus or bacterial or a combination of both. Bacterial tracheitis can evolve as a rare complication of influenza virus infection. Tracheitis and tracheobronchitis can cause airway obstruction as dry and thick sputum can block the airway.

Symptoms of bacterial tracheitis and tracheobronchitis include:

- Increased amount of thick mucus that may yellow, green, blood tingled, and foul smelling
- Redness, rash and/or inflamed at stoma site
- Bouts of deep barking cough, and high-pitched wheezing sound
- Fever
- Congested lung sounds
- Increased respiratory effort or change in respiratory rate
- Listlessness

Bacterial tracheitis can be a medical emergency especially in a laryngectomee and may require hospitalization. It may require intense respiratory tract care, fluid management, and antimicrobial therapy.

Treatment of tracheitis and tracheobronchitis is challenging in laryngectomees. It require special care of the stoma which includes clearing the thick sputum and the crusting around it which can compromise breathing. (See the table above in the **Bronchitis Section**).

Whenever antimicrobial therapy is given it should be guided by the results of the cultures of the tracheal secretion. Symptomatic treatment includes taking antipyretics, antitussive drugs, expectorants and mucolytics.

The risk of acquiring these infections can be reduced by:

- Getting vaccinated for the pneumococcal bacteria and the influenza viruses.
- Consult your physician about getting vaccinated for *Haemophilus influenzae* and *Neisseria meningitidis*
- Washing one's hands before any stoma care
- Wearing an HME
- Maintaining adequate respiratory tract humidification
- Avoiding hypothermia and breathing cold air

Caring for a runny nose and blowing the nose

Because laryngectomees and other neck breathers no longer breathe through their nose their nasal secretions are not being dried by moving air. Consequently the secretions drip out of the nose whenever large quantities of them are produced. This is especially common when one is exposed to cold and humid air or irritating smells. Avoiding these conditions can prevent a runny nose.

Wiping the secretion is the best practical solution. Laryngectomees using a voice prosthesis may be able to blow their nose by occluding the tracheostoma and divert air through the nose. There are several methods by which blowing the nose is possible for laryngectomees. Because the nose remains connected to the mouth swallowing saliva produces sufficient suction to pull down mucus from the nose which are subsequently swallowed.

An alternative method is to sniff and blow the nose by using the air pressure generated by moving the tongue backward and forward while it touches the top of the mouth while the lips stay closed. Blowing the nose, is done one nostril at a time. This requires occluding one nostril at a time by placing a finger on its side.

Other methods include: gently cleaning each nostril the with a voice prosthesis brush by twirling it around inside the nostril; those with voice prosthesis can occlude their stoma and forcefully exhale while the mouth is closed one nostril at a time; using a suction bulb to collect the secretion.

Keeping the nose secretion thin makes it easier to blow the nose. This can be achieved by being well hydrated and breathing humidified air or placing saline drops in the nose.

Respiratory rehabilitation

After a laryngectomy the inhaled air bypasses the upper part of the respiratory system and enters the trachea and lungs directly through the stoma. Laryngectomees therefore lose the part of the respiratory system that used to filter, warm and humidify the air they breathe.

The change in the way breathing is done also effects the efforts needed to breathe and potential lung functions. This requires adjustment and retraining. Breathing is actually easier for laryngectomees because there is less air flow resistance when the air bypasses the nose and mouth. Because it is easier to get air into the lungs, laryngectomees no longer need to inflate and deflate their lungs as completely as they did before. It is therefore not unusual for laryngectomees to develop reduced lung capacity and breathing capabilities.

There are several measures available to laryngectomees that can preserve and increase their lung capacity:

- The use of a HME can create resistance to air exchange. This forces the individual to fully inflate their lungs to get the needed amount of oxygen.

- Regular exercise under medical supervision and guidance. This can get the lungs to fully inflate and improve individuals' heart and breathing rates.
- Using diaphragmatic breathing. This method of breathing allows for greater utilization of the lung capacity.

Another problem is the sensation of shortness of breath that some laryngectomees develop when they exercise. Normally people exhale hard when exercising. However, they propel air out against the resistance of their vocal cords, which prevents collapse of the bronchial tubes. Exhalation of air in a laryngectomee is easier and quicker as they do not have cords that modify the exhalation. Because they can no longer control their exhalation, the deflation of their bronchi generates a sensation of shortness of breath. Although an HME can generate some back pressure it is not adjustable in a physiological fashion.

Laryngectomees who also suffer from chronic obstructive pulmonary disease (COPD) may find that maintaining their lung capacity is more difficult as they cannot fully inflating their lungs because of lack of pressure from their nose and mouth.

Chapter 8:

Stoma care in laryngectomees

A stoma is an opening that connects a portion of the body cavity to the outside environment. (**Picture 2**) A stoma is created after a laryngectomy to generate a new opening for the trachea in the neck, thus connecting the lungs to the outside. Caring for the stoma to insure its patency and health is crucial.

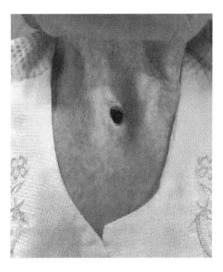

Picture 2: Stoma.

General care

It is very important to cover the stoma at all times in order to prevent foreign material (i.e., dirt, dust, smoke, bugs) from getting into the trachea and lungs.

There are various kinds of stoma covers. The most effective ones are called Heat/Moisture Exchangers (HME) because they create a tight seal around the stoma. In addition to filtering dirt, HMEs preserve some of the moisture and heat inside the respiratory tract and prevent the person from losing them. The HME therefore assists in restoring the temperature, moisture and cleanliness of the inhaled air to the condition before the laryngectomy.

The stoma often **shrinks** during the first weeks or months after it is created. To prevent it from closing completely, a tracheostomy or laryngectomy tube is initially left in the stoma 24 hours a day. Over time this duration is gradually reduced. It is often left overnight until there is no more shrinking. A laryngectomy tube is a soft, silicone tube that fits into the stoma. Those with inadequate stoma (too small, too large or deformed) may benefit from surgical repair (stomaplasty).

Stoma care when using a base plate or adhesive housing: The skin around the stoma can become irritated (i.e., red, inflamed) because of repeated gluing and removal of the housing. The materials used to remove the old housing and prepare for the new one can irritate the skin. The removal of the old housing can also irritate the skin especially when it is glued.

An adhesive removal wipe containing liquid (e.g., Remove ™, Smith & Nephew, Inc. Largo Fl 33773) can assist in removing the base plate or housing. It is placed at the edge of the housing and helps the housing detach from the skin when it is lifted off. Wiping the area with Remove ™ cleans the site from remnants of seal used to glue the housing. It is important to wipe off the leftover Remove ™ with an alcohol wipe so that it will not irritate the skin. When a new housing is use, wiping off the Remove ™ prevents it from interfering with placing glue again.

It is generally not recommended to leave the housing on for more than 48 hours. Some individuals, however, keep the housing much longer, and replace it when it becomes loose or dirty. In some people the removal of the adhesive is more irritating than the adhesives. In the event the skin is irritated, it is better to leave the housing on only for 24 hours. If the skin is irritated, it may be advisable to give the skin a rest for a day or until the area heals and cover the stoma only with a rigid base without any glue or with a foam cover. There are special hydrocolloid adhesives that allow use on sensitive skin.

It is important to use liquid film-forming skin protecting dressing (i.e., Skin Prep™ Smith & Nephew, Inc. Largo Fl 33773) before placing the glue.

Stoma care when using tracheostomy tube: The buildup of mucus and the rubbing of the tracheostomy tube can irritate the skin around the stoma. The skin around the stoma should be cleaned at least twice a day to prevent odor, irritation and infection. Using a hydrocolloid adhesive is often a good solution for patients with sensitive skin.

If the area appears red, tender or smells bad, stoma cleaning should be performed more frequently. Contacting one's physician is advisable if a rash, unusual odor, and/or yellowish-green drainage appear around the stoma. This may represent a bacterial infection.

Do and don't in stoma care:

- **Keep the stoma clean:** Keep the inside of the stoma clean, moist, and glistening. Saline "bullets" can help keeping it moist.
- **Use a clean face cloth** to clean the stoma.
- **Avoid using cotton balls or paper tissues to clean the stoma**: These may get sucked into your breathing tube or trachea and cause breathing problems.
- **Keep the tracheostomy tube clean:** *If you wear a tube follow your physicians and nurses* direction for its care.
- **Cover stoma at all times:** Use a heat and moisture exchanger (HME), gauze, cotton, or crocheted covers.
- **Do not use cotton or cotton-filled gauze to clean:** The fibers may get sucked into your trachea.
- **Exercise with moderation:** Excessive whenever you can but without too much strain.
- **Dress comfortably:** Allow for circulation of air, coughing and protection of clothing from coughing and secretions.
- **Cover stoma when coughing or sneezing:** Use thick paper tissues or handkerchiefs to pick up any coughed mucus.

- **Wear identification:** Carry medical identification. It is available from the American Cancer Society, Medic Alert and or your physician.
- **Have regular medical examinations:** Have regular examinations with your primary and ear nose and throat physicians.
- **Do not allow water to enter your stoma:** Do not swim unless you use a Larchel snorkel, which helps protect your airways. Use care in bathing, shaving. Use a shower shield or a moist towel to cover your stoma.
- **Do not inhale smoke, dirt, dust or irritating fumes:** Avoid inhaling smoke, dust or irritating fumes, and use stoma covers to protect you from inhaling insects or objects.

Cleaning the stoma

These are the general guidelines for keeping the airways and stoma clean:

- The area around the stoma and inside the wall of the trachea should be regularly checked for accumulated mucus and crusts in the morning, before going to sleep, and a throughout the day. A good source of light (i.e., flashlight) and a mirror to view the stoma are essential.
- Gently wash the skin around the opening with a clean face cloth and mild soap and water and wipe it dry. Keeping the stoma and the skin around it clean and free from secretions, can prevent skin irritation.
- It is important to humidify the inhaled air. This prevent stoma crusting, eases breathing, and reduces coughing. Wearing a stoma cover (i.e., HME) helps keep your stoma clean, dust free, and retains moisture.
- If there is mucus in the stoma it can be coughed or suctioned (using suction machine) out. Using saline bullets, saline spray, inhaling water steam (i.e., humidifier), can help in expelling the mucus by making it less viscous.

- The inside of the stoma and the voice prosthesis (TEP) can be cleaned using cotton-tipped swabs and blunt tweezers. This should be done using good lighting and a mirror. Caution is needed to prevent injuring the trachea in the cleaning process.

Skin irritation around the stoma

If the skin around the stoma becomes irritated and red, it is best to leave it uncovered (after cleaning it gently with non-allergenic soap and water) by a base plate and HME and not expose it to any solvents for a while (an hour to 2 days) so that it can heal. Sometimes individuals can develop an irritation to some of the solvents used to prepare and glue an HME base plate (housing). Avoiding these solvents and finding others that do not cause irritation is helpful.

Some individuals with sensitive skin that may prone to skin irritation may benefit from a skin friendly base plate such as OptiDerm™ (Atos Medical) which is made of a hydrocolloid material.

If signs of infection such as open ulcers and redness are evident, topical antibiotics can be useful. Seeking advice from one's physician is helpful especially if the lesion does not heal. The physician can obtain a bacterial culture of the affected area that can guide the choice of antimicrobial therapy.

Protecting the stoma from water when showering

It is important to prevent water from entering the stoma when taking a shower. A small amount of water in the trachea generally does not cause any harm and can be rapidly coughed out. However, inhalation of a large amount of water can be dangerous.

Methods to prevent water from entering the stoma are:

- Covering the stoma with the palm and not inhaling air when water is directed at the vicinity of the stoma.

- Wearing a bib with the plastic side out.(**Picture 3**)

- Using a commercial device that covers the stoma. (**Picture 4 & 5**)

- Wearing one's stoma cover, the base plate or HME housing while showering may be sufficient especially if water flow is directed away from the stoma.

- Pausing air inhalation for a few seconds while washing the area close to the stoma is also helpful.

- Taking a shower at the end of the day just before removing the HME and its housing is a way to use the housing for water protection. This simple method can make taking a shower easier.

- Some individuals can learn to take a shower without protecting their stoma using the lowest water stream. This can be done by either facing the shower head, or bending the chin to cover the stoma. Alternatively one can turn their back to the shower head and tilt their head backward allowing the water to reach the hair from behind.

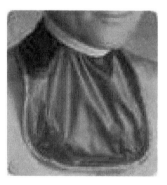

Picture 3: Wearing a bib.

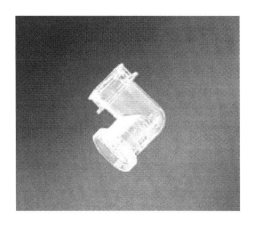 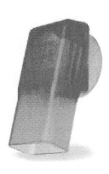

Picture 4: InHealth Stoma Shower Device   **Picture 5: Provox (Atos Medical) ShowerAid**

Water inhalation and aspiration pneumonia

Aspiration pneumonia is rare in laryngectomees because they cannot aspirate saliva from their mouth as their lungs are not connected to the mouth. However, aspiration pneumonia can develop when bacteria get into the lungs from the stoma's area and cannot be expelled out by coughing. This can occur when the mucus is not adequately coughed out usually because it is too dry. Maintaining mucus with clear consistency is imperative (See **Chapter 7**).

It is also very important to cover the stoma at all times in order to prevent bacteria and viruses from getting into the trachea and lungs. Cleaning one's hands before touching the stoma or the HME can reduce the risk of introducing bacteria and viruses to the lungs.

Laryngectomees are at risk of inhaling (aspirating) water that may not be free of bacteria. Taking a bath is not recommended for laryngectomees because of the risk of water aspiration. Those who take a bath should keep the water level up to their hips when seated.

Tap water contains bacteria; the number of bacteria varies, depending on the cleaning efficacy of the water treatment facilities and their source (e.g., well, lake, river etc.). Pool water contains chloride that reduces, but never sterilize the water. Sea water contains numerous bacteria; their nature and concentrations varies.

When unclean water or non-sterile saline gets into the lungs it can sometimes cause pneumonia. Developing aspiration pneumonia depends on how much water is inhaled and how much is coughed out, as well as on the individuals' immune system.

Swimming as a laryngectomee

Swimming or getting into water can be very dangerous for laryngectomees. Once the stoma is under water, water can gets into the trachea and the lungs leading to drowning. This can also cause aspiration pneumonia. It may be safe to wade in shallow and calm water as long as the water level is kept at a safe distance below the stoma to enable breathing and avoid aspiration.

Some laryngectomees take short swims or get under the water for a few seconds after occluding their stoma with a finger. Some wear a baseplate and seal it with an improvised locked HME.

There may be emergency situations where a laryngectomee is forced to get into the water. In such situation it is advisable to:

- Keep the stoma above water level
- Avoid breathing (for a short time) when the water gets into the stoma
- Wear a life vest that keeps the stoma above water level
- Use a floating device that lifts the body as much as possible

It is advisable that laryngectomees avoid situations that may put them at risk of getting into water such as rafting, canoeing. When planning a boat ride or cruise it would be wise to:

- Have a life vest available and floating tube (with automatic, non-manual inflation)
- Wear your life vest when needed
- Be aware of the evacuation routes and locations of floating devices and lifeboats

- Practice evacuation procedures
- Inform others and the cruise staff of your special needs

Some life vests and floating devices require manual air inflation. Since laryngectomees are unable to do that, they may choose to carry a small air pump to inflate the devices.

Some special devices have been created to allow neck breathers to swim. The Larchel snorkel is a rubber device-a breathing tube inside an inflatable cuff is inserted into the stoma and then inflated with an air syringe, forming a seal. It is available in Europe and requires a physician's prescription and training.

The risks involved in swimming and diving are high. Neck breathers should consult their physicians and speech and language pathologist before attempting to swim.

Preventing aspiration of tissue or paper into the stoma

One of the major causes of respiratory emergency in a neck breather is the aspiration of tissue or paper towels into their trachea. This can be very dangerous and cause asphyxiation. It usually happens after covering the stoma with a paper towel when coughing out sputum. Following the cough there is a very deep inspiration of air that can suck the paper back into the lungs. The way to prevent this is to use a cloth towel or a strong paper towel that does not break easily, even when moist. Thin tissues should be avoided.

Another way to prevent aspiration of paper tissues is to hold one's breath until one has completely finished wiping off the sputum and removed the paper tissue or paper towel from the stoma area.

Aspiration of other foreign material should also be prevented by covering the stoma at all times by an HME, foam cover, or stoma cover.

Aspiration of water into the stoma while taking a shower can be prevented by wearing a device that covers the stoma (see above). One can keep the HME on while showering and/or avoid breathing in when water is directed at the stoma's site.

Taking a bath in a tub can be done safely as long as the water level does not reach the stoma. The areas above the stoma should be washed with a soapy washcloth. It is important to prevent soapy water from entering the stoma.

Covering (hiding) the Stoma and HME

Following laryngectomy, individuals breathe through a tracheostomy site that opens through a stoma on their neck. Most place an HME or a foam filter over the stoma to filter the inhaled air and maintain warmth and humidity in the upper airways. The covered stoma site is prominent, and laryngectomees face a choice whether to cover the HME or filter with a garment, an ascot, or jewelry or to leave it uncovered.

The pros and cons of each choice are:

Breathing may be easier without an additional cover which can interfere with air flow. Leaving the area exposed allows for easier access to the stoma for purpose of cleaning and maintenance and enables a rapid removal of the HME in case one needs to cough or sneeze. The urge to cough or sneeze is often very sudden and if the HME is not taken out quickly it can become clogged with mucus.

Exposing the site provides an unspoken explanation for the weak and rusty voice of many laryngectomees and encourages others to listen to them more attentively. It also makes it easier for health care providers to recognize the laryngectomee's unique anatomy in case emergency respiratory ventilation is needed. If this condition is not rapidly recognized ventilation may be administered through the mouth or nose rather than through the stoma.

Openly displaying the covered stoma site also reveals the person's medical history and the fact that he/she are cancer survivors who go on with their lives despite their handicap, cancer being the leading indication for a laryngectomy. Although there are many cancer survivors in the community, their identity is hidden from outward appearances.

Those who cover their stoma site with a stoma cover or cloth often do it because they do not want others to be distracted or offended by the site. They also do not want to expose anything that is disfiguring and want to be inconspicuous and appear as normal as possible. Covering the site is often more common among females who may be more concerned with their physical appearance. Some individuals feel that being a laryngectomee is only a small part of who they are as a person; and they do not want to "advertise" it.

There are advantages and repercussions to each approach and the final selection is up to the individual.

Chapter 9:

Heat moisture exchanger (HME) filter care

Heat and Moisture Exchanger (HME) filter serve as stoma covers and create a tight seal around the stoma. In addition to filtering dust and other larger airborne particles, HMEs preserve some of the moisture and heat inside the respiratory tract and prevent their loss, and adds resistance to the airflow. HME filters assist in restoring the temperature, moisture and cleanliness of the inhaled air to the same condition as before laryngectomy.

HME advantages

It is very important that laryngectoees wear an HME. In the United States the filters are available through Atos Medical and InHealth Technologies. The HME filter can be attached by using an intraluminal device inserted into the trachea or stoma, that includes laryngectomy or tracheostomy tubes, Barton Mayo Button™ and/or Lary Button™. The filter can also be inserted into a housing or a base plate attached to the skin around the stoma.

The foam media captures the warm, moistened, and humidified air upon exhalation. It is impregnated with chlorhexidine (anti-bacterial agent), sodium chloride (NaCl), calcium chloride salts (traps moisture), activated charcoal (absorbs volatile fumes), and is disposable after 24 hours of use.

HME cassettes are designed to be removed and replaced on a daily basis. (**Picture 6**) The foam media in the cassettes are treated with agents that have antimicrobial properties and help to retain moisture in the lungs. They should not be washed and reused because these agents lose their effectiveness over time or when rinsed by water or other cleaning agents.

The filter's advantages also include: increasing the moisture within the lungs (subsequently leads to less mucus production), decreasing the viscosity of the airway secretions, decreasing risk of mucus plugs, and re-instating the normal airway resistance to the inhaled air which preserves the lung capacity.

In addition, the HME filters reduce the inhalation of bacteria, viruses, dust and pollen. Inhaling less pollen can reduce the airway irritation during high allergens season. Wearing HME may reduce the risk of getting viral and bacterial infection, especially in crowded or closed places.

Laryngectomees with breathing problems such as chronic obstructive pulmonary disease (COPD), emphysema, asthma, etc., should consult their physicians before trying HME.

A new HME filter that is combined with an electrostatic filter is designed to filter potential respiratory pathogens (Provox Micron TM, Atos Medical). This HME most closely resemble the normal nasal properties, as it does not only conditions, but also filters the inhaled air, and also filters the exhaled air. The electrostatic filter eliminates transfer of particulate material and airborne organisms from and to the laryngectomized patient.

It is important to realize that simple stoma covers, such as a laryngofoam TM filter, ascot, bandana, etc., do not provide the same benefits as a HME filter.

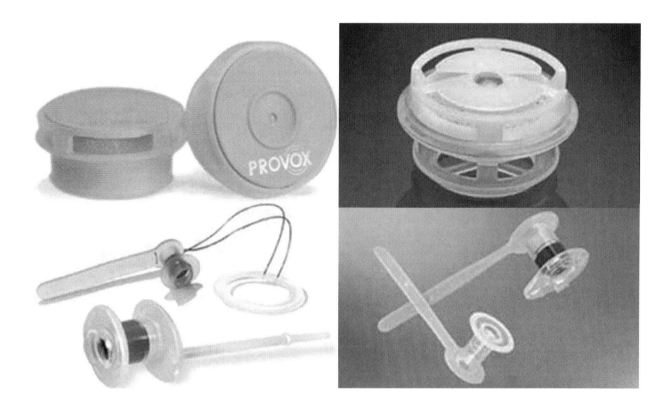

Picture 6: Voice prosthesis (below) and HMEs (above) produced by Atos Medical (Provox) and InHealth.

Cleaning mucous from the HME

It is normal for laryngectomee to cough and clear secretions throughout the day. With continued use of an HME, these secretions generally become more manageable. Many individuals notice that the amount of their secretions diminishes and become less thick. This does not occur overnight and several weeks may be required to notice this change.

When the HME is used right after laryngectomy there is not much adjustment needed, because up to the surgery the nose and throat were still functioning. However, when the laryngectomee starts using an HME not right away after the surgery, it takes time to adjust to it. This is because air resistance with the HME is higher than that with an open stoma breathing, and some patients may feel some discomfort. This can be avoided by starting with a lower resistance HME and switching after a few days up to a week to a regular resistance HME.

More mucus is initially produced by laryngectomee after starting using an HME, when this is not done after the operation. This is because the airways of these individuals got used to produce more mucus and moisture which were lost during exhalation. These vapors are captured by the newly worn HME and the laryngectomee experiences retention of more mucus. This generally last a few days until the airways adjust to the effects of the HME.

When mucous is coughed, it will rest against the back of the HME cassette were plastic bars known as "mucous guards" are preventing the mucous from deeply penetrating the foam. When this happens, it may become difficult to breathe until the mucous is cleared. It is important, therefore, to wipe off the mucous from the HME cassette (using a soft cloth, a tissue, or a dedicated soft toothbrush) as often as necessary to ensure one is breathing comfortable and their secretions are well managed. When adequate cleaning is not possible the HME should be replaced.

The effect of an HME on breathing of a laryngectomee

Laryngectomy compromises the respiratory system by allowing the inhaled air to bypass the nose and upper airways which normally provide humidification, filtration and warmth. It also reduces the resistance and the effort needed for inhalation by removing air resistance and shortening the distance the air travels to their lung. This means that laryngectomees do not have to work as hard to get air past the upper part of the system (nose, nasal passages, and throat), and their lungs do not have to inflate as much as they did before unless the person works to retain their capacity through exercise and other methods. An HME increases the resistance to inhaled air and therefore increases inhalation efforts, thus preserving previous lung capacity and function.

When needing extra air (i.e., running, biking) the HME can be temporarily removed and the stoma can be covered by cloth. There are less restrictive HMEs that offer less resistance to air passage and allow greater air flow (i.e., Atos Medical's XtraFlow). These type of HME can be used when exercising and when adapting to the breathing resistance after having been without an HME for a longer time.

Placing an HME housing (including base plate)

The key to prolonging the use of an HME's housing is not only properly gluing it in place, but also removing the old adhesives and glue from the skin, cleaning the area around the stoma and applying new layers of adhesive and glue.

In some individuals the shape of the neck around the stoma makes it difficult to fit a housing or a base plate. There are several types of housing; and a speech and language pathologist (SLP) can assist in selecting the best one. Finding the best HME housing may take trial and error. Over time, as the post-surgical swelling subsides and the area around the stoma reshapes itself, the type and size of the housing may change.

The buildup of mucus at the bottom of the base plate can weaken the adhesion of the base plate and eventually cause the base plate seal to break leading to air leak. The accumulation of mucus in the space behind the base plate can be minimized by placing the base plate (housing) as down as possible attaining the maximum distance between the stoma and bottom part of the seal. This allows the mucus a longer way to travel before getting to the bottom, which would then give more time to remove the mucus before it caused the base plate to fail. Because the anatomy of the stoma and the skin around it is unique for each person, finding the best location for placing the base plate can be guided by one's SLP or otolaryngologist.

Below are the suggested instructions on how to place the housing for the HME. (**Picture 7**) Throughout the process it is important to wait patiently and allow the liquid film-forming skin protecting dressing (i.e., Skin Prep™ Smith & Nephew, Inc. Largo Fl 33773)" and silicone skin adhesive to dry before applying the next item or placing the housing. This takes time, but it is important to follow these instructions:

1. Clean the old glue with an adhesive removal wipe (e.g., Remove ™, Smith & Nephew, Inc. Largo Fl 33773).
2. Wipe off the Remove ™ with an alcohol wipe. (if not wiped off Remove ™ will interfere with the new adhesive).
3. Wipe the skin with a wet towel.
4. Wipe the skin with the wet towel with soap. Clean any debris, dry mucus, and dirt. Remove any hair.
5. Wash away the soap with a wet towel and thoroughly dry.
6. Apply Skin Prep™ and let it dry for 2-3 minutes.
7. For extra adhesion apply Silicone Glue (Atos Medical) or Skin-Tac TM wipe (Torbot, Cranston, Rhode Island 20910) and let it dry for 3-5 minutes. The Silicon Glue provides extra adhesion which is important for users of a hands free HME.
8. Use one hand to stretch the skin around the stoma to smooth it as much as possible. Use the other hand to attach the housing for the HME at the best location to allow air flow and good attachment. Attempt to place it as down as possible attaining the maximum distance between the stoma and bottom part of the seal. Press the ring firmly to the skin making sure it is glued also to any deep creases or seams in the skin.
9. When using hands free HME wait for 25-30 minutes before speaking to allow the adhesive to "set".

Some SLPs recommend warming the housing prior to placement by rubbing it in the hands, holding it under the armpit for a few minutes, or by blowing warm air on it with a hair drier. Be careful that the adhesive does not become too hot. Warming the adhesive is especially important when you use a hydrocolloid adhesive since the warmth activates the glue.

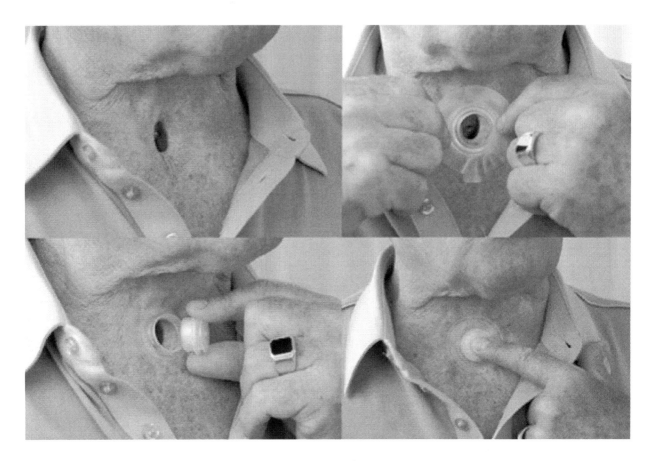

Picture 7: Placement of HME and its base plate (housing) on a stoma.

Using Provox® LaryButton™ or Barton-Mayo Button™

Provox®LaryButton™ and Barton-Mayo Button™ are an alternative solution to using adhesive housing for those who are using an HME filter,/or hands-free valve but who experienced various problems including losing the seal or allergic reactions to the glue. The buttons provide leak proof tracheostoma valve retention for near-total laryngectomy and total laryngectomy patients.

They are constructed from soft silicone material and no traumatically shaped to reduce negative side-effects such as stoma irritation and bleeding. (**Pictures 8 & 9**) They can be worn by laryngectomees regardless of their speaking method. The Provox® LaryButton™ has LaryClips to support retention of the LaryButton, especially when using an automatic speaking valve like the FreeHands HME.

Using the Button requires that the stoma be pretty regular in shape (circular), and have regular and even surfaces on both sides of the stoma. However, there are some alterations which a clinician can make to the Button to compensate for some irregular stoma surfaces. It is also possible to get the Buttons custom made for the contours of an individual stoma. The HME filters from both ATOS and InHealth fit the Buttons.

The buttons can be used only in those whose voice prosthesis lumen is not blocked by them. The proper insertion and use of the Buttons should be taught and practiced with the assistance and guidance of SLP or one's otolaryngologist.

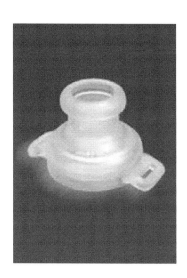

Picture 8: Provox®LaryButton™

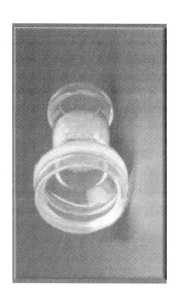

Picture 9: Barton-Mayo Button™

Using hands free HME

The hands free HME allows speaking without the need to manually press on the HME to close it off thus blocking exhalation through the stoma and directing air to the voice prosthesis. This device frees one's hand and eases vocational and recreational possibilities. Note that when using a hands free HME more pressure is generated when air is exhaled, thus potentially leading to a break in the HME housing's seal. Reducing the exhalation pressure when speaking, speaking slower and softly (almost whispering), and taking a breath after 4-5 words can prevent a break in the seal. Supporting it with a finger before needing to speak loud can also help. It is also important to quickly remove the device before coughing.

Several hands free devices are commercially available. Atos Medical offers the Provox® FreeHands HME™ and the new Provox® FreeHands Flexivoice™. InHealth Technologies markets the Adjustable Tracheostoma Valve II (ATSV II.)® (see pictures below). (**Pictures 10 & 11**) All devices enable automatic occlusion. The new Provox FreeHands Flex® allows both automatic and manual occlusion and a choice between a moist or high air flow HMEs.

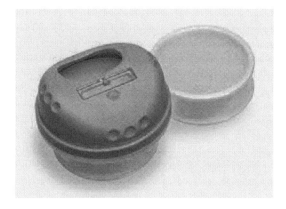

Picture 10: Atos Medical Provox® FreeHands Flexivoice™

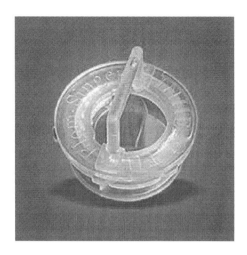

Picture 11: InHealth Technologies Adjustable Tracheostoma Valve II (ATSV II.)®

The air filter (also called cassette in Provox FreeHands HME) for the hands free device has to be changed on a regular basis (every 24 hours or sooner if it becomes dirty or covered with mucus). However, the HME device can be used for 6 months to a year. Proper use and cleaning can prolong its life. The hands free device requires initial adjustments to fit the laryngectomee's breathing and speaking abilities. Detailed instructions on how to use and care for the devices are provided by their manufacturers.

Meticulously following the instructions how to place a base plate (see above) helps in maintaining the ability to speak using a hands free HME without breaking the baseplate's seal.

The key to speaking with a hands free HME is to learn how to speak without breaking the seal. Using diaphragmatic breathing allows for more air to be exhaled, thus reducing speaking efforts and increasing the number of words that can be articulated with each breath. This methods prevents buildup of air pressure in the trachea which can break the base plate's seal. It may take time and patience to learn how to speak in such a way, and guidance by a skilled SLP can be helpful.

Speech can be made clearer and easier by:

- Speaking slowly
- Speaking only 4-5 words between each air exhalation

- Using diaphragmatic breathing
- Over articulating the words
- Speaking by using low air pressure

Laryngectomees often try to compensate for their low volume by increasing the exhalation air pressure. This is tiring and can lead to air leak around the HME's base plate.

It is very important to place the HME housing according to the steps outlined in the section on HME care (see "Placing an HME Housing" above) including cleaning the area around the stoma with Remove ™ alcohol, water and soap, placing Skin Prep TM and finally glue (Skin Tag ™). Following these instructions can prolong the life of the HME housing and reduce the likelihood of an air leak through the seal.

Air inhalation is slightly more difficult when using a free HME as compared to a regular HME. It is possible to allow for greater amounts of air intake by rotating the valve counter-clockwise in Atos FreeHands ™ , Atos Medical Provox® FreeHands Flexivoice™ and InHealth HandsFree ™ devices. In situation where greater exchange of air is needed it may be useful to temporarily replace the hands free HME with a regular one, or to temporarily remove it .The hands free device should be used only when awake. It should be cleaned on a regular basis and when it get clogged with mucus according to the manufacturers' instructions.

Challenges using hands free HME: Patients who have difficulty achieving and/or maintaining a reliable seal may not be successful in using a hands free HME. This is particularly true if the shape of the neck around the stoma is irregular because of extensive surgery, reconstruction, etc.

Excessive "back pressure" can make using a hands free HME very difficult. Back pressure refers to the amount of pressure generated while transferring air from the lungs through the pharynx and out of the mouth. Those who develop back pressure feel as if they have to "push" somewhat to talk. The buildup of pressure is exerted against the device and the adhesive housing, which will lead to breaking of the seal. Some causes of excessive back pressure can be treated effectively. Training and guidance by the SLP can help in optimizing one's speaking ability and ensure the lowest level of back pressure possible.

Despite the challenge of keeping the seal, many laryngectomee value the ability to speak in a more natural way and the freedom of using both hands. Some learn that they can keep the seal much longer when they use a voice amplifier, thus requiring less effort and generating less air pressure.

Wearing the HME overnight

Some HMEs are approved for wear 24/7 (i.e., Provox^R Luna; Atos Medical) is designed to be worn at nighttime by offering low breathing resistance.(**Picture 12**) It has side openings designed to prevent occlusion while sleeping. It is made of hydrogel that soothes the skin during the nighttime.

The advantage of wearing the HME 24/7 is that its beneficial effects are extended throughout the whole day. A hands free HME should be replaced by a regular HME cassette when sleeping.

If the seal lasts, one can keep it overnight. If it does not, it is possible to use an improvised base plate for the night period. An Atos Xtra BasePlate^{TM} can be trimmed by removing the outer soft part and leaving the inner rigid part. The plate is "sticky" and thus can cover the stoma without glue, even enabling one to speak. It is also possible to use the HME inserted in a LaryTube overnight.

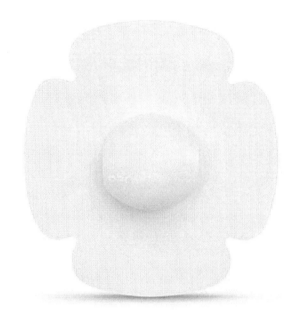

Picture 12: Provox Luna

HME and housing care during radiation treatment

RT directed at the area around the stoma does not harm or effect the voice prosthesis. RT can cause inflammation and easy bleeding and crusting of the trachea during treatment and recovery periods. This is why it may be difficult for laryngectomies to use the voice prosthesis (TEP) during that time. It is, however, important to continue to clean the prosthesis.

Wearing an HME allows the laryngectomee to continue to benefit from its advantages. However, wearing adhesive HME housing is not recommended as the skin around the stoma usually become inflamed. An alternative method for housing during the treatment and recovery periods is to use a LaryTube. The SLP can guide and assist in choosing the best method for housing of the HME.

Chapter 10:

Tracheo-esophageal voice prosthesis use and care in laryngectomees

Restoring speech communication using a voice prosthesis was a significant medical advancement for laryngectomees. It enables the laryngectomee to create sound again immediately after its insertion. A voice prosthesis is inserted through a previously created tracheoesophageal puncture (TEP) connecting the trachea and esophagus in those wishing to speak through tracheo-esophageal speech. It enables the individual to exhale pulmonary air from the trachea into the esophagus through a silicone prosthesis that connects the two; the vibrations are generated by the lower pharynx.

Types of voice prosthesis

There are two types of voice prosthesis: an indwelling one that is installed and changed by a speech and language pathologist (SLP) or otolaryngologist and a patient-changed one.

The indwelling prosthesis generally lasts a longer time than the patient managed device. However, prosthesis eventually leak mostly because yeast and other microorganisms grow into the silicone leading to incomplete closure of the valve flap. When the valve flap does not close tight anymore, fluids can pass through the voice prosthesis (see below in Causes of voice prosthesis leak section).

An indwelling prosthesis can function well for weeks to months. However, some SLPs believe that it should be changed even when it does not leak after six months because, if left for a longer time, it can lead to dilatation of the puncture.

The patient managed voice prosthesis allows greater degree of independence. It can be changed by the laryngectomee on a regular basis (every 1-2 weeks). Some individuals change the prosthesis only after it starts leaking. The old prosthesis can be cleaned and reused several times.

A number of factors determine an individual's ability to use a patient managed prosthesis:

- The location of the puncture should be easily accessible; the site of the puncture may, however, migrate over time, making it less accessible.
- The laryngectomee should have adequate eyesight and good dexterity, enabling him/her to perform the procedure, and capable of following all the steps involved. An indwelling voice prosthesis does not need to be changed as frequently as a patient managed one.

The main difference between the clinician-changed and patient-changed voice prosthesis is the size of the flanges. The larger size flanges on the clinician-changed devices make it harder to accidentally dislodge it. Another difference is that the insertion strap should not be removed from the patient-changeable prosthesis because its helps to anchor the prosthesis. There is generally no difference in voice quality between a clinician-changed and a patient-changed device.

Potential contra-indications for having voice prosthesis

Not every laryngectomee is able to use voice prosthesis. Relative contra indications for voice prosthesis include:

- Poor dexterity
- Poor eye sight

- Poor pulmonary function

- Impaired mental status

- Lack of motivation

- Inability to manage associated care of stoma and voice prosthesis

- Voicing difficulties

- Recurrent aspiration and dislodging of the TEP

- Difficulty in occluding the stoma

- Proximity of speech pathologist or otolaryngologist

- Lack of support system

- Potential cost and lack of reimbursement

What to do if the prosthesis leaks or is dislodged

If the prosthesis leaks or has become dislodged or has been removed accidentally, a patient-changed prosthesis can be inserted by those who carry an extra device. Alternatively, a red rubber catheter can be inserted into the TEP which can close within a few hours, to prevent closure. Inserting a catheter or a new prosthesis can prevent the need for a new TEP. Leakage of the prosthesis from the center (lumen) can be temporarily handled by inserting a plug (specific to the type and width of the prosthesis) until it can be changed. It is therefore advisable that individuals using voice prosthesis carry a prosthesis plug and catheter.

Dislodging of the TEP usually occurs when patients attempt to clean or replace the device and a cough is stimulated. Sudden inspiratory effort increases the risk of aspirating the device when it is not secure at the trachea. When the TEP is dislodged, one of three possibilities may occur:

- The patient may cough it out.
- It may fall into the esophageal side of the fistula tract and get swallowed where it will eventually pass through the digestive tract.

- It may fall into the trachea and become aspirated. This will immediately generate intense coughing that may expel the prosthesis though the stoma. If this occurs the patient must seek medical attention immediately, as this can be life-threatening. It is important to have the inhaled prosthesis removed from the lungs.

The most common location for device impaction is at the level of the upper right main stem bronchus and carina. This usually is well tolerated, but an uncomfortable shortness of breath (dyspnea) is present. Because of the potential lethal consequences of an aspirated prosthesis, it should always be considered and evaluated whenever a prosthesis is lost.

Causes of voice prosthesis leak

There are two patterns of voice prosthesis leak-leak through the prosthesis and leak around it.

Leakage **through the voice prosthesis** is predominantly due to situations in which the valve can no longer close tightly. This may be due the following: colonization of the valve by fungus; the flap valve may get stuck in the open position; a piece of food, mucus or hair (in those with a fee flap) stuck on the valve; or the device coming in contact with the posterior esophageal wall. Inevitably, all prostheses will fail by leaking through, whether from Candida colonization or simple mechanical failure.

If there is continuing leakage through the prosthesis from the time it is inserted, the problem is generally caused by the flap's valve remaining open because of negative pressure generated by swallowing. This can be corrected by using a prosthesis that has a greater resistance. The trade-off is that having such a voice prosthesis may require more effort when speaking. It is nevertheless important to prevent chronic leakage that can lead to aspiration into the lungs.

Leakage **around the voice prosthesis** is less common and is mainly due to TEP tract dilation or the inability to grip the prosthesis. It has been linked to shorter prosthesis life time. It may occur when the puncture, that houses the prosthesis widens. During insertion of the voice prosthesis, some dilation of the puncture takes place, but if the tissue is healthy and elastic, it should shrink back after a short time. The inability to contract back can be associated with gastroesophageal reflux, poor nutrition, alcoholism, hypothyroidism, improper puncture placement, incorrectly fitted prosthesis, TEP tract trauma, local granulation tissue, recurrent or persistent local or distant cancer, past radiation treatment and radiation necrosis.

Leakage around the prosthesis can also occur if the prosthesis is too long for the user's tract. Whenever this occurs, the voice prosthesis moves back and forth in the tract (pistoning) thereby dilating the tract. The tract should be measured and a prosthesis of more appropriate length should be inserted. In this circumstance leakage should resolve within 48 hours. If the tissue around the prosthesis does not heal around the shaft within this time period, comprehensive medical evaluation is warranted to determine the cause of the problem.

Another cause of leakage around the prosthesis is the presence of narrowing (stricture) of the esophagus. The narrowing of the esophagus forces the laryngectomee to swallow harder, with greater force so that the food/liquid goes through the stricture. The excess swallowing pressure pushes the food/liquid around the prosthesis.

Several procedures have been used to treat persistent leakage around the prosthesis. These include temporary removal of the prosthesis and replacement with a smaller-diameter catheter to encourage spontaneous shrinkage; using customized prostheses; placing a purse-string suture around the puncture; injection of gel, collagen or micronized AlloDerm® (LifeCell, Branchburg, N.J. 08876); cautery with silver nitrate or electrocautery; autologous fat transplantation; inserting a larger prosthesis to stop the leak, and surgical or non-surgical (removing the prosthesis allowing closure to occur) closure of the puncture. Treatment of reflux (the most common cause of leakage) can allow the esophageal tissue to heal. Granulation tissue can be removed by cauterization (electro-, chemo-, laser-).

Increasing the diameter of the prosthesis is generally not recommended. Generally a larger diameter TEP is heavier than a smaller one, and the weakened tissue is often not able to support a bigger device, making the problem even worse.

Some, however, believe that using a larger diameter prosthesis reduces the speaking pressure (larger diameter allows better airflow) which allows greater tissue healing to occur while when the underlying cause (most often reflux) is treated.

The use of a prosthesis using a larger esophageal and/or tracheal flange may be helpful, as the flange acts as a washer to seal the prosthesis against the walls of the esophagus and/or trachea, thus preventing leakage.

Both types of leakage can cause excessive, strenuous, coughing which may even lead to development of abdominal wall and inguinal hernias. The leaked fluid can enter the lungs, causing aspiration pneumonia. Any leakage can be confirmed by direct visualization of the prosthesis while drinking colored liquid. If leakage occurs and cannot be corrected after brushing and flushing the voice prosthesis, it should be changed as soon as possible.

With the passage of time, a voice prosthesis generally tends to last longer before it begins to leak. This is because the swelling and increased mucus production are reduced as the airways adapt to the new condition. Improvement is also due to better prosthesis management by laryngectomees as they familiarize themselves with their device.

Patients with a TEP need to be followed by an SLP because of normal changes in the tracheo-esophageal tract. Re-sizing of the tract may be needed as it can change in length and diameter with time. The length and diameter of the prosthesis' puncture generally change over time as the swelling generated by creation of the fistula, surgery and radiation gradually decreases. This require repeated measurements of the length and diameter of the puncture tract by the SLP who can select a properly sized prosthesis.

One of the advantages of having a voice prosthesis is that it can assist in dislodging food stuck in a narrow throat. When food get stuck above the prosthesis, trying to speak or blowing air through the voice prosthesis can sometimes force the stuck food upward and relieve the obstruction.

The prosthesis may have to be changed if there is an alteration in the quality of the voice especially when the voice becomes weaker or one needs more respiratory effort to speak. This may be due to yeast growth which interferes with the opening of the valve.

What to do if the indwelling voice prosthesis leaks

Persistent leakage of the voice prosthesis into the trachea induces cough especially when liquids are ingested. The leakage carries several risks which include:

- Development of aspiration pneumonia
- Clogging of HME
- Social embarrassment
- Anxiety
- Temporary increase of blood pressure and pulse
- Avoiding food and liquid intake causing dehydration and weight loss
- Emergence of inguinal hernia
- Urinary incontinence (involuntary leakage of urine)

A leak can take place when a piece of dry mucus, a food particle, or hair (in those with a free flap) prevents a complete closure of the prosthesis's valve. Cleaning the prosthesis by brushing and flushing it with warm water (see previous section) can remove these obstructions and stop the leakage.

If the leakage through the voice prosthesis happens within three days after its insertion it may be due to a defective prosthesis or one that was not placed correctly. It takes some time for the yeast to grow. If the prosthesis leaks when new, it is due to another cause. In addition to brushing and flushing with warm water, cautiously rotating the prosthesis a couple of times to dislodge any debris may help. If the leak persists the voice prosthesis should be replaced.

The easiest way of temporarily stopping the leak until the voice prosthesis can be changed is use a plug. A plug is specific for the type and width of each voice prosthesis. It is a good idea to obtain a plug from the prosthesis' manufacturer and have it handy. Sealing the prosthesis will prevent speaking but it allows eating and drinking without leakage. The plug can be removed after eating and drinking and reinserted as needed. Some individuals use a small cotton swab inserted into the prosthesis lumen to absorb the leaking fluid. This method runs the risk of dropping the swab into the trachea. These are temporary solutions until the voice prosthesis is replaced.

It is important to stay well hydrated despite the leakage. Avoiding fluid losses in hot weather through perspiration by staying in an air-conditioned environment and ingesting liquids in a way that is less likely to leak are helpful. Speaking while drinking can reduce or even prevent the liquids to leak inside the trachea. Drinks that contain caffeine increase urination and should be avoided..

Viscous (thickened) fluids tend not to leak and consuming them can provide essential liquids despite the leak. Many food items that contain large amount of liquids are more viscous (i.e., jelly, soup, oat meal, toast dipped in milk, yogurt) and are therefore less likely to leak through the prosthesis. On the other hand coffee and carbonated drinks are more likely to leak. Fruits and vegetables (e.g., watermelon, apples, etc.) contain large amount of water. The way to find out what works is to cautiously try any of these.

Another method to reduce the leak until the prosthesis can be changed which may work for some individuals is to try and swallow the liquid as if it is a food item. Such maneuver is less likely to lead to fluid leakage through the voice prosthesis.

These measures can be used to keep well-hydrated and nourished until the voice prosthesis can be changed.

Cleaning the voice prosthesis and preventing leaking

It is very important to keep the voice prosthesis clean to insure their proper function and durability. When not cleaned properly the prosthesis can leak, and the ability to speak can be compromised or weakened. It is recommended that the voice prosthesis be cleaned at least twice a day (morning and evening), and preferably after eating because this is the time when food and mucus can become trapped. Cleaning is especially helpful after eating sticky foods or whenever one's voice is weak. A prosthesis cleaning brush and flushing bulb are used in cleaning the prosthesis.

It is advisable to clean the voice prosthesis' inner lumen at least twice a day and after each meal. Maintenance and prevention of leakage guidelines are:

1. Before using the brush provided by the manufacturer (**Picture 13**), dip it in a cup of hot water and leave it there for a few seconds.
2. Insert the brush into the prosthesis (not too deep) and twist it around a few times to clean the inside of the device.
3. Take the brush out and rinse it with hot water and repeat the process 2-3 times until no material is brought out by the brush. Because the brush is dipped in hot water one should be careful not to insert it beyond the voice prosthesis inner valve to avoid traumatizing the esophagus with excessive heat.
4. Flush the voice prosthesis twice using the bulb provided by the manufacturer (**Picture 14**) using warm (not hot!) potable water. To avoid damage to the esophagus sip the water first to make sure that the water temperature is not too high.
5. Prevent yeast growth (see below)

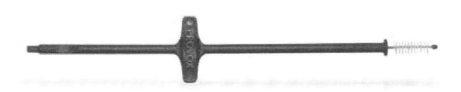

Picture 13: A voice prosthesis cleaning brush (Atos Medical)

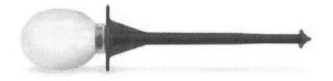

Picture 14: A voice prosthesis flushing bulb (Atos Medical)

Warm water works better than room temperature water in cleansing the prosthesis probably because it dissolves the dry secretions and mucus and perhaps even flushes away (or even kills) some of the yeast colonies that had formed on the prosthesis.

Initially the mucus around the prosthesis should be cleaned using tweezers preferably with rounded tips. Following that the manufacturer-provided brush should be inserted into the prosthesis and twisted back and forth. The brush should be thoroughly washed with warm water after each cleaning. The prosthesis is then flushed twice with warm (not hot) water using the manufacturer's provided bulb.

The flushing bulb should be introduced into the prosthesis opening while applying slight pressure to completely seal off the opening. The angle that one should place the tip of the bulb varies between individuals. (The SLP can provide instructions how to choose the best angle.) Flushing the prosthesis should be done gently because using too much pressure can lead to splashing of water into the trachea. If flushing with water is problematic, the flush can also be used with air.

The manufacturers of each voice prosthesis brush and flushing bulb provide directions of how to clean them and when they should be discarded. The brush should be replaced when its threads become bent or worn out.

The prosthesis brush and flushing bulb should be cleaned with hot water, when possible, and soap and dried with a towel after every use. One way to keep them clean is to place them on a clean towel and expose them to sunlight for a few hours, on a daily basis. This takes advantage of the antibacterial power of the sun's ultraviolet light to reduce the number of bacteria and fungi.

Placing 2-3 cc of sterile saline (**Picture 15**) in the trachea at least twice a day (and more if the air is dry), wearing an HME 24/7 and using a humidifier can keep the mucus moist and reduce the clogging of the voice prosthesis.

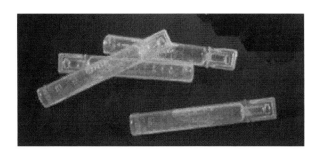

Picture 15: A sterile saline vial for respiratory tract use ("Saline bullet")

Preventing yeast growth in the voice prosthesis

Overgrowth of yeast is one cause of a voice prosthesis leaking and thus failing. Nevertheless, it takes some time for yeast to grow in a newly installed voice prosthesis and form colonies that prevent its valve's from closing completely. Accordingly, failures immediately after voice prosthesis installation are unlikely due to yeast growth.

The presence of yeast should be established by the person who changes the failing voice prosthesis This can be done by observing the typical yeast (Candida) colonies that prevent the valve from closing and, if possible, by sending a specimen from the voice prosthesis for fungal culture.

Mycostatin (an antifungal agent) is often used to prevent voice prosthesis failure due to yeast. It is available with a prescription in the form of a suspension or tablets. The tablets can be crushed and dissolved in water. There is anecdotal information that apple cider vinegar that is known to inhibit candida growth can be used to gargle and be swallowed to prevent yeast growth on the TEP.

Automatically administering anti-fungal therapy (i.e., mycostatin) just because one assumes that yeast is the cause of voice prosthesis failure may be inappropriate without proof. It is expensive, may lead to the yeast developing resistance to the agent, and may cause unnecessary side effects.

There are, however, exceptions to this rule. These include the administration of preventive anti-fungal agents to diabetics; those receiving antibiotics; chemotherapy or steroid; and those where colonization with yeast is evident (coated tongue etc.).

There are several methods that help prevent yeast from growing on the voice prosthesis:

- Reduce the consumption of sugars in food and drinks, brush your teeth well after consuming sugary food and/or drinks.
- Brush your teeth well after every meal and especially before going to sleep.
- Clean your dentures daily.
- Diabetic should maintain adequate blood sugar levels.
- Take antibiotics and corticosteroids only if they are needed.
- After using an oral suspension of an antifungal agent, wait for 30 minutes to let it work and then brush your teeth. This is because some of these suspensions contain sugar.
- Dip the voice prosthesis brush in a small amount of mycostatin suspension or vinegar and brush the inner voice prosthesis before going to sleep. (A homemade suspension can be made by dissolving a quarter of a mycostatin tablet in 3-5 cc water). This would leave some of the suspension inside the voice prosthesis. The unused suspension should be discarded. Do not place too much mycostatin or vinegar in the prosthesis to prevent dripping into the trachea. Speaking a few words after placing the suspension will push it towards the inner part of the voice prosthesis.
- Consume probiotics by eating active-culture yogurt and/or a probiotic preparation.
- Gently brush the tongue if it is coated with yeast (white plaques)
- Replace the toothbrush after overcoming a yeast problem to prevent re colonizing with yeasts
- Keep the prosthesis brush clean

The use of probiotics such as Lactobacillus acidophilus to prevent yeast overgrowth

A probiotic that is often used to prevent yeast overgrowth is a preparation containing the viable bacteria Lactobacillus acidophilus. There is no FDA approved indication to use *Lactobacillus acidophilus* to prevent yeast growth. This means that there were no controlled studies to ensure its safety and efficacy. *L. acidophilus* preparations are sold as a nutritional supplement and not as a medication. The recommended dosage of *L. acidophilus* is between 1 and 10 billion bacteria. Typically, acidophilus tablets contain somewhere within this recommended amount of bacteria. Dosage suggestions vary by the tablet's brand, but generally it is advised to take between one and three *L. acidophilus* tablets daily.

Although generally believed to be safe with few side effects, oral preparations of *L. acidophilus* should be avoided in people with intestinal damage, a weakened immune system, or with overgrowth of intestinal bacteria. In these individuals this bacterium can cause serious and sometimes life threatening complications. This is why individuals should consult their physician whenever this live bacteria is ingested. It is especially important in those with the above conditions.

Chapter 11:

Upper airway issues after laryngectomy: Eating, swallowing, belching, esophageal dilatation, smelling, gastroesophageal reflux, fistula, and phonation problems

Eating, swallowing, and smelling are not the same after laryngectomy. This is because radiation and surgery create permanent lifelong changes. RD can cause fibrosis of the muscles of mastication which can lead to one's inability to open the mouth (trismus or lockjaw), making eating more difficult.

During laryngectomy, certain structures in the throat important in the natural act of swallowing are removed. Physically, swallowing is very different, since reconstruction can limit movement of the tongue base, important in driving food downward towards the esophagus. Additionally, with the removal of the vocal cords and the diverting of the trachea, subglottic pressure to drive food down the esophagus no longer exists, so the throat muscles have to handle more of the work.

Eating and swallowing difficulties can also be generated by a decrease in the production of saliva, and a narrowing of the neopharynx (new pharynx) and esophagus, plus the lack of peristalsis in those with flap reconstruction. Swallowing difficulties and painful swallowing can lead to accumulation of saliva and oral secretion in the mouth. Smelling is affected because inhaled air bypasses the nose.

This chapter describes the manifestations and treatment of the eating and smelling challenges faced by laryngectomees. These include swallowing problem, food reflux, esophageal strictures, and smelling difficulties.

Maintaining adequate nutrition and liquid consumption in a laryngectomee

Eating may be a lifelong challenge for laryngectomees. This is because of swallowing difficulties, decreased production of saliva (which lubricates food and eases mastication), and an alteration in one's ability to smell.

The need to consume large quantities of fluid while eating can make it difficult to ingest large meals. This is because when liquids fill the stomach there is little room left for food. Because liquids are absorbed within a relatively short period of time, laryngectomees end up having multiple small meals rather than fewer large ones. The consumption of large quantities of liquid makes them urinate very frequently throughout the day and night. This can interfere with one's sleep pattern and can cause tiredness and irritability. Those who suffer from heart problems (e.g., congestive heart failure) may experience problems due to overloading their bodies with excess fluid.

Consuming food that stays longer in the stomach (e.g., proteins such as white cheese, meat, nuts) can reduce the number of daily meals, thus reducing the need to drink liquids.

It is important learn how to eat without ingesting excessive amounts of liquid. Relieving swallowing difficulties can reduce the need to consume fluids, while consuming less liquids prior to bedtime can improve sleeping pattern.

Nutrition can be improved by:

- Ingesting adequate but not too much liquid
- Drinking less liquid in the evening
- Consuming "healthy" food
- Consuming a low carbohydrate and high protein diet (high sugar enhances yeast colonization)
- Requesting dietitian assistance

It is essential to make sure a laryngectomee follows an adequate and balanced nutrition plan that contains the correct ingredients, despite difficulties with their eating. A low carbohydrate and high protein diet that includes vitamins and minerals supplements is important. The assistance of a nutritionist, speech and language pathologist (SLP), and physicians in ensuring that one maintains adequate weight is very helpful.

How to remove (or swallow) food stuck in the throat or the esophagus

Some laryngectomees experience recurrent episodes of food becoming stuck in the back of their throat or esophagus and preventing them from swallowing.

Clearing the stuck food can be accomplished using these methods:

1. First do not panic. Remember that you cannot suffocate because as a laryngectomee, your esophagus is completely separate from your trachea.
2. Try to drink some liquid (preferably warm) and attempt to force the food down by increasing the pressure in your mouth. Sometimes changing the position of the head while swallowing to the right or left allows the stuck food to be move down into the stomach. If this does not work-
3. If you speak through a tracheo-esophageal voice prosthesis try to speak forcefully. This way, the air you blow through the voice prosthesis may push the food above it into the back of your throat, relieving the obstruction. Try this first standing up and if it does not work bend over a sink and try to speak. If this does not work-
4. Bend forward (over a sink or hold a tissue or cup over your mouth), lowering your mouth below the chest and applying pressure over your abdomen with your hand. This forces the contents of the stomach upward and may clear the obstruction.

These methods work for most people. However, everyone is different and one needs to experiment and find the methods that work best for them. Swallowing does, however, get better in many laryngectomees over time.

Some laryngectomees report success in removing the obstruction by gently massaging their throat, walking for a few minutes, jumping up on their feet, sitting and standing several times, hitting their chest or the back, using a suction machine with the catheter paced in the back of their throat, or just waiting for a while until the food is able to descend into the stomach on its own.

If nothing works and the food is still stuck in the back of the throat it may be necessary to be seen by an otolaryngologist or go to an emergency room to have the obstruction removed.

How to swallow and avoid food from getting stuck in the esophagus or throat

Swallowing as a laryngectomee requires patience and care. Following an episode of food obstruction in the upper esophagus swallowing may be difficult for a day or two. This is probably because of the local swelling in the back of the throat; normally, this will disappear with time.

Ways to avoid such episodes:

- Eating slowly and patiently
- Taking small bites of food and chewing very well before swallowing
- Swallowing a small amount of food at a time and always mixing it with liquid in the mouth before swallowing. Warm liquid makes it easier to swallow.
- Moisten dry/crumbly foods with sauces, gravies, olive oil, margarine, or butter.
- Some food items (soft diet items) are easier to swallow: soup, yogurt, blended food, ice cream, banana, etc.

- Moisten dry/crumbly foods with sauces, gravies.
- Flushing the food with more liquids as needed. (Warm liquids may work better for some individuals in flushing down the food)
- Sit upright while eating/drinking, and stay upright for at least 30-45 minutes after mealtime
- Avoiding food that is sticky or hard to chew.

One needs to find out for him/her self what food is easier to ingest. Some foods are easy to swallow (e.g., toasted or dry bread, yogurt, and bananas) and others tend to be sticky (e.g., unpeeled apples, lettuce and other leafy vegetables, and steak).

Swallowing tablets and capsules

Ingestion of large pills and capsules may be difficult for laryngectomees. Over time, laryngectomees generally learn the maximal size of pills and capsules that they can swallow.

Tips to take medications include:

- Some medications are available in several dosages which may be manufactured in smaller size pills or capsules. It is therefore possible to swallow the desired dose by taking several small pills or capsules.
- The size of pills of some generic medications may vary depending on their manufacturers. If this is the case it may be possible to find a smaller size pill produced by a different manufacturer.
- Some medications are also available as a suspension. It is best to check with one's physician and pharmacy if a commercially available suspension is available, or can be prepared by one's pharmacy.

- Pills can be crushed and dissolved in room temperature liquids, or broken down to small pieces prior to ingestion. However, slow release medications may lose their time delay action when crushed. Ingestion of large gel capsules may not be possible.

- Capsules can be opened and their content swallowed. However, this exposes some medication to the stomach acidity that may inactivate and reduce their potency.

- Some crushed medications or capsule contents may be irritating to the mouth and/or esophagus and stomach. Take them with food and flush them with liquids.

- It is best to check with one's physician and/or pharmacist if dissolving a pill or capsule's contents is an option.

- When oral ingestion is not an option other routes of drug administration may be possible. These include intramuscular and intravenous injection, aerosols, and rectal or vaginal suppositories.

- When the size of a tablet or capsule is too large the physician may select a similar medication (from the same class or with similar effects) that is available in smaller size pill or capsule.

Belching (burping), hiccup and air trapping in laryngectomees

Laryngectomees are prone to develop burping and hiccup especially in the immediate period after surgery. One cause for this is that the post-surgical narrowing of their upper esophagus may interfere with the upward passage of swallowed air which is collected in the esophagus and stomach. These issues may persist in many individuals.

Air trapping below the esophageal narrowing is common in those who use voice prosthesis where some of the air directed to the esophagus can collect. Also rapid swallowing of food and liquids (gulping) can allow excessive air to collect in the esophagus and stomach. One may also swallow excess air when talking while eating, chewing gum, sucking on hard candies, drinking carbonated beverages, or smoking.

Acid reflux or gastroesophageal reflux disease (GERD) can sometimes cause excessive belching by promoting increased swallowing. Chronic belching may be caused by inflammation of the stomach lining (gastritis) or an infection with *Helicobacter pylori*, the bacteria that can cause stomach ulcers. In these cases, the belching is accompanied by other symptoms, such as heartburn or abdominal pain. Poorly fitting dentures can cause excess air swallowing when eating and drinking. Belching may be enhanced by foods that relax the lower esophageal sphincter, such as chocolate, fats, and mints.

The most common symptoms of excessive air swallowing (aerophagia) is belching, hiccups, bloating, abdominal pain, abdominal distension, and flatulence.

Excessive air swallowing can be reduced by:

- Eating and drinking slowly
- Chewing the food well
- Eating and drinking in the upright position
- Avoiding speaking while eating or drinking
- Avoiding chewing gum, sucking on hard candies, drinking carbonated beverages (including beers), or smoking
- Treating esophageal narrowing (i.e., dilatation) (see below)
- Speaking slowly with low air pressure when using voice prosthesis

The collected air can also trigger hiccups. A hiccup is an involuntary, spasmodic contraction of the diaphragm and intercostal muscles that results in sudden inspiration. Hiccups are usually caused by gastric distention from overeating, swallowing air, drinking carbonated beverages.

Hiccups can be treated by physical maneuvers and medications.

The physical maneuvers include:

- Holding one's breathing

- Moderately forceful attempted exhalation against a closed airway, usually done by closing one's stoma, while pressing out as if blowing up a balloon (Valsalva maneuver)
- Swallowing granulated sugar, hard bread, or peanut butter
- Breathing into a paper bag
- Gargling cold water
- Drinking from opposite side of glass
- Stimulating of nasooropharynx with a cotton swab
- Pulling on the tongue
- Biting on a lemon
- Pulling ones knees to chest or leaning forward to compress the chest

Speaking when eating after laryngectomy

Laryngectomees who speak through a tracheo-esophageal voice prosthesis may have difficulties in speaking when they swallow. This is especially challenging during the time it takes the food or liquids to pass by the esophageal voice prosthesis site. Speaking during that time is either impossible or sounds "bubbly". This is because the air introduced into the esophagus through the voice prosthesis has to travel through the food or liquids. Unfortunately it takes the food much longer to go through the esophagus, especially in someone who had had a flap to replace the pharynx. This is because that flap has no peristalsis (contraction and relaxation) and the food goes down mainly due to gravity.

It is therefore important to eat slowly, mix the food with liquids while chewing and allow the food to pass through their voice prosthesis area before trying to speak. Over time, laryngectomees can learn how much time is needed for food to pass through the esophagus to allow speaking. It is helpful to drink before attempting to speak after eating.

There are eating and swallowing exercises that a SLP can teach a laryngectomee that may assist them in relearning how to swallow without difficulties.

Swallowing difficulties

Laryngectomees are usually not allowed to swallow food immediately after surgery and must be fed through a feeding tube for 2-3 weeks. The tube is inserted into the stomach through the nose, mouth or the tracheo-esophageal puncture and liquid nourishment is supplied through the tube. This practice, however, is slowly changing; there is increasing evidence that in standard surgeries, oral intake can start with clear liquids as soon as 24 hours after surgery. This may also help with swallowing as the muscles involved with continue to be used.

Most laryngectomees experience problems with swallowing (dysphagia) immediately after their surgery. Because swallowing involves the coordination between more than 20 muscles and several nerves, damage to any part of the system by surgery or radiation can produce swallowing difficulties. The majority of laryngectomees relearn how to swallow with minimal problems. Some may only need to make minor adjustments in eating such as taking smaller bites, chewing more thoroughly, and drinking more liquids while eating. Some experience significant swallowing difficulties and may require assistance in learning how to improve their ability to swallow by working with an SLP who specializes in swallowing disorders. Swallowing dysfunction, due to fibrosis often requires a change in diet, pharyngeal strengthening, or swallow retraining especially in those who have had surgery and/or chemotherapy. Swallowing exercises are increasingly used as a preventing measure.

Swallowing function change after a laryngectomy and can be further complicated by radiation and chemotherapy. The incidence of swallowing difficulty and food obstruction can be as high as 50% of patients and, if not addressed, can lead to malnutrition. Most difficulties with swallowing are noticed after discharge from the hospital. They can occur when attempting to eat too fast and not chewing well. They can also happen after trauma to the upper esophagus by ingesting a sharp piece of food or drinking very hot liquid. These can cause swelling which may last a day or two.

Patients experience difficulties in swallowing (dysphagia) as a result of:

- Abnormal function of the pharyngeal muscles (dysmotility)

- Cricopharyngeal dysfunction of the cricoid cartilage and the pharynx
- Reduced strength of the movements of the base of the tongue
- Development of a fold of mucous membrane or scar tissue at the tongue base called "pseudoepiglottis". Food can collect between the pseudoepiglottis and the tongue base
- Difficulty with tongue movements, chewing, and food propulsion in the pharynx because of removal of the hyoid bone and other structural changes
- A stricture within the pharynx or esophagus may decrease food passage leading to its collection
- Development of a pouch (diverticulum) in the pharyngoesophageal wall that can collect fluid and food resulting in the complaint of food "sticking" in the upper esophagus

The free flap that is sometimes used to replace the larynx has no peristalsis, making swallowing even more difficult. After surgery in such cases food descends to the stomach mostly by gravity. The time for the food to reach the stomach varies between individuals and ranges from 5 to 10 seconds.

Chewing the food well and mixing it with liquid in the mouth prior to swallowing is helpful, as is swallowing only small amounts of food each time and waiting for it to go down. Drinking liquids between solid foods is helpful in flushing down the food. Eating takes longer; one must learn to be patient and take all the time needed to finish the meal.

The swelling that develops after surgery tends to decrease over time, which reduces the narrowing of the esophagus and ultimately makes swallowing easier. This is good to remember because there is always hope that swallowing will improve within the first few months after surgery. However, if this does not occur dilatation of the esophagus is one of the therapeutic option. Dilatation is usually done by an otolaryngologist or gastroenterologist (see below in the Dilatation of the esophagus section).

In most cases, dilation is successful, and the patients stabilizes within six weeks to eight months. A small number of patients, however, continue to have severe dysphagia. Temporary placement of nonmetal expandable stents can be effective for managing refractory benign strictures. If the problem persists pharyngeal reconstruction may be needed. This can be accomplished by obtaining a flap of non-radiated tissue (i.e., forearm) to create a wider throat.

Tests used for the evaluation of swallowing difficulty

There are five major tests that can be used for the evaluation of swallowing difficulties:

- Barium swallow radiography
- Videofluoroscopy (motion X-ray study)
- Upper endoscopic evaluation of swallowing
- Fiberoptic nasopharyngeal laryngoscopy
- Esophageal manometry (measures esophagus muscle contractions)

The specific test is chosen according to the clinical condition.

Videofluoroscopy which is usually the first test done to most patients, records swallowing during fluoroscopy. (**Picture 17**) It allows accurate visualization and study of the sequence of events which make up a swallow; it is limited to the cervical esophagus. The video, taken from both the front and the side, can be viewed at a slower speeds to enable accurate study. This helps identify abnormal movement of food, such as aspiration, pooling, movement of anatomic structures, muscle activities, pharyngeal constrictor spasm, pharyngoesophageal stricture, and exact oral and pharyngeal transit times. The effects of various barium consistencies and positions can be tested. Thick or solid food boluses can be used for patients who complain of solid food dysphagia.

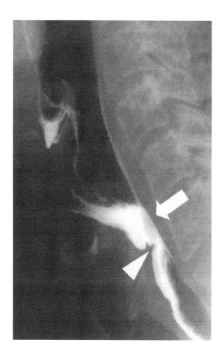

Picture 17: Esophageal videofluoroscopy (arrow shows stricture)

Narrowing (strictures) of the neopharynx and esophagus

A stricture of the esophagus is a narrowing along the pharyngo-esophagus that blocks or inhibits the ease of food passage, resulting in the esophagus having an hour-glass configuration.

Strictures after laryngectomy can be due to the effects of radiation as well as the tightness of the surgical closure and can also occur gradually as scarring develops.

Interventions that can help the patient include:

- Dietary or postural changes
- Myotomy (cutting the muscle)
- Dilatation (see below)
- Placement of self-expanding plastic stents (see below)

Alternatives to these procedures include nasal enteric tubes, gastrostomy tubes, and jejunostomy tubes. Total parenteral nutrition can also be used in patients who are not candidates for these therapeutic options.

Esophageal stents

An esophageal stent is a flexible mesh tube, approximately 2cm (3/4 inch) wide, and is placed through the constricted area of the esophagus to allow food and beverages to pass from the mouth to the stomach. The stent is not as wide or as flexible as a normal esophagus and care must be taken not to block it while eating.

Stent placement usually requires both endoscopic and fluoroscopic guidance, but can be done with either modality safely. In general, dilation of a stricture before placing the stent is not required. Most stents are placed distally and across the gastroesophageal junction, but proximal stent placement (which requires more precise placement) can also be performed. (**Picture 18**) Complications include bleeding and perforation (which are rare) as well as migration, tumor overgrowth, and tumor ingrowth (which are more common).

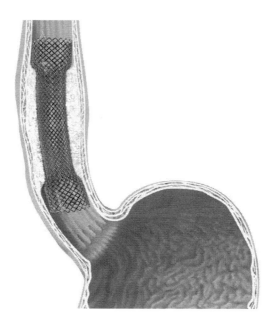

Picture 18: Esophageal stent in place

Dilatation of the neopharynx and esophagus

Narrowing of the neopharynx (the surgically reconstructed new pharynx) and esophagus is a very common consequence of radiation treatment as well as laryngectomy; and dilatation of the esophagus is often needed to reopen it. The procedure usually needs to be repeated and the frequency of this procedure varies among individuals. In some people this is a lifelong requirement and in others the neopharynx and esophagus may stay open after a few dilatations. The procedure requires sedation or anesthesia because it is painful. A series of dilators with greater diameter are introduced into the esophagus to dilate it slowly. (**Picture 19**) While the process breaks down the fibrosis, the condition may return after a while.

Sometimes a balloon rather than a long dilator is used to dilate a local stricture. Another method that may help is the use of topical and or injectable steroids to the esophagus. Although dilation is done by an otolaryngologist or a gastroenterologist, in some cases it can be accomplished by

173

the patient at home by performing self-dilations at-home device. In difficult cases, surgery may be needed to remove the stricture or replace the narrow section with a graft (tissue flap).

Because dilation breaks down fibrosis, the pain generated by the procedure may last for a while. Taking pain medication can ease the discomfort.

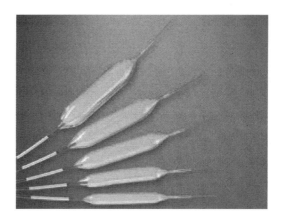

Picture 19: Wire Guided Balloons used for esophageal dilatation

Voicing problems when using tracheoesophageal speech

Laryngectomees using tracheoesophageal speech can develop a strained, halted or aphonic voice. These difficulties can be due to pharyngeal constrictor spasm, post-operative edema (swelling), inappropriate occlusion of the stoma, voice prosthetic issues, and pharyngoesophageal stricture.

Pharyngeal constrictor spasm or pharyngeal hypertonicity: Pharyngeal constrictor spasm occurs when the patient attempts to voice and the pharynx responses by tightens to prevent or limit airflow up through the vibratory segment. This can result in no sound (complete closure of the pharynx with spasm); a brief sound followed by no sound (immediate release of air followed by complete closure of the pharynx with spasm); or a strained vocal quality (partial closure of the pharynx with spasm). In almost all instances this is not something that develops over time and a laryngectomee will either have this issue post-operatively or will not.

Post-operative edema: Swelling of the tracheoesophageal walls following surgery can narrow and even close the vibratory segment of the pharyngoesophagus and cause voicing issues similar to when pharyngeal constrictor spasm is present. Voicing difficulties dissipate over time as the edema subsides.

Inappropriate occlusion of the stoma when voicing: How a patient occludes the stoma for voicing can alter the quality of his/her voice. Digital occlusion with an incomplete seal will lead to a weaker voice quality with turbulent air escape further compromising intelligibility. Too much pressure with digital occlusion can compress the vibratory segment and cause hypertonicity or complete inability to speak (aphonia). If excessive digital pressure during occlusion is the issue, patient training of light touch for occlusion is all that is needed.

Voice prosthetic issues affecting voicing: There are several factors related to the voice prosthesis that can cause a voice quality that mimics that of pharyngeal constrictor spasm. A prosthesis that is partially or completely clogged by dried mucus can cause a strained voice or inability to speak. Removing the mucus will eliminate the issue and enable normal voicing.

An inappropriately-fitted voice prosthesis can also cause similar vocal difficulties. A voice prosthesis that is too long may press against the esophageal wall reducing or preventing airflow through the device. A voice prosthesis that is too short may result in narrowing of the esophageal side of the tracheoesophageal tract causing a strained voice or aphonia. Voice prosthetic issues can be ruled out by removing the voice prosthesis, making sure the appropriate sized dilator can pass easily through the tracheoesophageal tract and testing the vocal quality once the dilator is removed through an open tract. If the voicing difficulty persists with open tract voicing prosthetic issues have been ruled out.

Swallowing difficulties as a cause of voicing problems: Difficulty or inability to swallow solids, may be due to blockage of the swallowing tube caused by a stricture. Dilatation of the neopharynx and esophagus (see above) can improve phonation. However, this may require repeated dilatations as narrowing may recur.

Fluoroscopy is used to diagnose both pharyngeal constrictor spasm and pharyngoesophageal stricture when speaking and swallowing. Pharyngeal constrictor spasm appears as a transient bulge in the posterior pharyngeal constrictor muscles when attempting to speak. Stricture, however, is identified during swallowing and appears as a narrowing of the neopharynx or esophageal lumen as contrast material transits through them. These two conditions can also co-occur.

Identifying the exact underlying issue causing the laryngectomee's voice disturbances and appropriate intervention can allow the patient to achieve fluent tracheoesophageal voicing.

Use of Botox® for pharyngeal constrictor muscle spasm

Botox® is a pharmaceutical preparation of toxin A which is produced by *Clostridium botulinum*, an anaerobic bacteria that causes botulism, a muscle paralysis illness. The botulinum toxin causes partial paralysis of muscles by acting on their presynaptic cholinergic nerve fibers through the prevention of the release of acetylcholine at the neuromuscular junction. In small quantities it can be used to temporarily paralyze muscles for 3-4 months. It is used to control muscle spasms, excessive blinking, and for cosmetic treatment of wrinkles. Infrequent side effects are generalized muscle weakness and rarely even death. Botox® injection has become the treatment of choice for selected individuals to improve swallowing and tracheo-esophageal speech after laryngectomy.

For laryngectomees, Botox® has been used to reduce the hypertonicity and spasm of the vibrating segment, resulting in an esophageal or tracheoesophageal voice that requires less effort to produce. However, it is only effective for overactive muscles and may require the injection of relatively large doses into the spastic muscles. It can be used to relax muscle tightness in the lower jaw when one experience difficulties in swallowing. It cannot help conditions that are not due to muscle spasms, such as esophageal diverticula, strictures due to fibrosis after radiation, and scars and narrowing after surgery.

A pharyngeal constrictor muscle hypertonicity or pharyngoesophageal spasm (PES) is a common cause for tracheo-esophageal speech failure following laryngectomy. In almost all cases, this develops immediately after laryngectomy and not over time. Constrictor muscle hypertonicity can increase peak intra-esophageal pressure during speaking, thus interfering with fluent speech. It may also disturb swallowing by interfering with the pharyngeal transit of food and liquids.

Botox® injection can be carried out by otolaryngologists in the clinic. The injection can be done percutaneously or through an esophago-gastro-duodeno-scope. The percutaneous injection into the pharyngeal constrictor muscles along one side of the newly formed pharynx (neopharynx) is done just above and to the side of the stoma.

An injection through an esophago-gastro-duodeno-scope can be performed whenever a percutaneous injection is not feasible. This method is used in patients with severe post-radiation fibrosis, disruption of the cervical anatomy, and anxiety or inability to withstand a percutaneous injection. This method allows direct visualization and greater precision. The injection into the PES segment is often done by a gastroenterologist and is followed by gentle expansion by balloon massage to facilitate uniform distribution of the Botox®.

Pharyngo-cutaneous fistula

A pharyngo-cutaneous fistula is an abnormal connection between the pharyngeal mucosa to the skin. Typically a salivary leak develops from the pharyngeal area to the skin, indicating a breakdown of the pharyngeal surgical suture line. It is the most common complication after laryngectomy and usually occurs 7-10 days after the operation. The main causes leading to development of fistula is poor wound healing. Things such as too much tension on the wound, a wound infection after surgery, poor nutrition, continued use of alcohol and tobacco, and prior radiation are the usual things that lead to problems with wound healing and the formation of a fistula.

Most fistulae will heal on their own without additional surgery. Until that occurs external drainage may need to be established to keep secretions out of the stoma and an alternative method of feeding such as a percutaneous endoscopic gastrostomy (PEG) is used. Surgical repair is reserved for those fistulae which do not close on their own and those that pose some danger particularly to the stoma and the lungs.

The closure of the fistula can be evaluated by a dye test (such as ingestion of methylene blue which appears in the skin if the fistula is unobstructed) and/or by radiographic contrast studies.

Smelling after laryngectomy

Laryngectomees may experience difficulties with their sense of smell. This is despite the fact that regular laryngectomy surgery, does not involve nerves related to smell and the sense of smell or olfaction, remains intact. What has changed, however, is the pathway of airflow during respiration. Before a laryngectomy, air flows into the lungs through the nose and mouth. This movement of air through the nose allows for scents to be detected as they come in contact with the nerve endings in the nose responsible for the sense of smell.

After a laryngectomy, however, there is no longer an active air flow through the nose. This can be perceived as a loss of smell. Patients, however, can relearn how to smell, by closing their mouths and swallowing to create a vacuum that introduces air into the nose.

The "polite yawn technique" can also help laryngectomees regain their capacity to smell. This method is known as the "polite yawn technique" because the movements involved are similar to those used when one attempts to yawn with a closed mouth. Swift, downward movement of the lower jaw and tongue, while keeping the lips closed, will create a subtle vacuum, drawing air into the nasal passages and enabling the detection of any scent through the new airflow. With practice, it is possible to achieve the same vacuum using more subtle (but effective) tongue movements.

How to avoid unpleasant smells

One "advantage" of being a laryngectomee is the ability to avoid unpleasant smells or odors such as cigarette smoke. This is because all our air intake is through the stoma, while smelling is done through our nostrils. This can be achieved by preventing the noxious smell from reaching the nose by:

- Squeezing the nostrils with the fingers
- Placing a cotton ball in each nostril
- Wearing a surgical mask over the nose with or without a fitted piece of plastic

Chapter 12:

Medical problems in head and neck cancer: pain management, acupuncture, cancer spread, hypothyroidism, dizziness, constipation, gastroesophageal acid reflux, and prevention of medical errors

This chapter describes a variety of medical issues affecting laryngectomees and head and neck cancer patients.

Hypertension is discussed in **Chapter 3 (page 69)** and lymphedema in **Chapter 5 (page 84)**.

Pain management

General pain

Many cancer patients and survivors complain of pain. Pain can be one of the important signs of cancer and may even lead to its diagnosis. Thus, it should not be ignored and should be a sign to seek medical care. The pain associated with cancer can vary in intensity and quality. It can be constant, intermittent, mild, moderate or severe. It can also be aching, dull, or sharp.

The pain can be caused by a tumor pressing or growing into and destroying nearby tissues. As the tumor increases in size, it may cause pain by putting pressure on nerves, bones or other structures. Cancer of the head and neck can also erode the mucosa and expose it to saliva and mouth bacteria. Cancer that has spread or recurred is even more likely to cause pain.

Pain can result also from treatments for cancer. Chemotherapy, radiation and surgery are all potential source of pain. Chemotherapy can cause diarrhea, mouth sores, and nerve damage. Radiation of the head and neck may cause painful and burning sensations to the skin and mouth, muscle stiffness and nerve damage. Surgery also can be painful, may leave deformities and/or scars that take time to improve.

Cancer pain can be treated by various methods. Eliminating the source of the pain through radiation, chemotherapy, or surgery is best, if possible. However, if not possible, other treatments include pain medications, nerve blocks, acupuncture, acupressure, massage, physical therapy, meditation, relaxation, and even humor. Specialists in pain management can offer these treatments.

Pain medication can be administered as a tablet, dissolvable tablet, intravenously, intramuscularly, rectally or through a skin patch. Medication includes: analgesics (e.g., aspirin, acetaminophen), nonsteroidal anti-inflammatory drugs (e.g., ibuprofen), weak (e.g., codeine) and strong opioids (e.g., morphine, oxycodone, hydromorphone, fentanyl, methadone). Other medications include carbamazepine (an anticonvulsant), and gabapentin (a GABA analog).

All these medications have side effects (i.e., constipation with codeine), and should be taken under medical supervision.

Sometimes patients do not receiving adequate treatment for cancer pain. The reasons for this include doctors' reluctance to inquire about pain or offer treatments, patients' reluctance to speak about their pain, fear of addiction to medications, and fear of side effects.

Treating pain can both increase patients' well-being, as well as ease the hardship imposed on their caregivers. Patients should be encouraged to talk to their health care providers about their pain and seek treatment. Evaluation by a pain management specialist can be very helpful; all major cancer centers have pain management programs.

Recent research has shown positive results for acupuncture in controlling pain. However, studies in people with cancer are often too small and it is more difficult to be sure of their results.

Chronic head and neck pain

Chronic head or neck pain after treatment can be debilitating and occurs in about 15 % of patients. Shoulder and neck pain are particularly common in those who also underwent neck dissection. It can cause functional limitations and contribute to unemployment in survivors.

The condition can be treated with physical therapy and appropriate pain control. Medications such as gabapentin and carbamazepine may be prescribed. Pain management services for treatment with narcotics and behavioral therapy are important assets in management of chronic pain. Acupuncture can provide significant reductions in pain, shoulder dysfunction, and dry mouth in head and neck cancer patients after neck dissection. (See next section)

The American Society of Clinical Oncology released the first set of practice guidelines to help clinicians manage chronic pain in adults with cancer In July 2016. The guidelines addresses screening and comprehensive assessment, treatment and care options-including pharmacologic and non-pharmacologic interventions-and paid special attention to the risks and benefits associated with opioid use. The Guidelines can be found at:

http://ascopubs.org/doi/full/10.1200/JCO.2016.68.5206

Acupuncture in managing side effects of treatment of head and neck cancer

Acupuncture can help with some physical problems such as pain and feeling sick. It can also help to reduce symptoms such as anxiety and assists individuals in relaxing and improving their overall feeling of wellbeing.

Acupuncture works by stimulating nerves to release substances that can reduce symptoms. The substances can also change some of the body's functions, such as muscle tension. A number of the body's natural morphine like substances (endorphins) are released in the nervous system to relieve pain. Serotonin, a pain reliever that promotes a feeling of wellbeing, is also released by acupuncture.

There is no evidence that acupuncture helps in treating or curing cancer. It is, however, helpful in relieving some symptoms of cancer and the side effects of cancer treatment. It has sown to work in relieving chemotherapy related sickness, tiredness and cancer pain. It can be very successful in treatment of some cancer-related pain and in reducing narcotic use and thereby minimizing their side effects.

Needling a variety of trigger and painful points, percutaneous electrical nerve stimulation, and osteo-puncture, along with whole body energetic acupuncture support, are approaches available to the acupuncturist. The practitioner puts fine, stainless steel, and disposable needles in different trigger points in the patient's skin. Often, treatment starts with only a few needles but this may change depending on the response and the number of symptoms the patient manifests. The needles shouldn't cause pain but might generate a tingling sensation. They are usually left in place for 10 to 30 minutes.

The degree of beneficial results from acupuncture treatment depends on various clinical factors such as presenting symptoms, clinical staging, timing of the encounter in the course of the illness, and the areas of involvement.

Acupuncture is used to treat a wide range of pain conditions and some other symptoms.

Some of the condition that acupuncture can be helpful that relate to head and neck cancer include:

- Acute and chronic pain control
- Dry mouth after radiation
- Muscle spasms, tremors, tics, contractures
- Peripheral neuropathy (also after chemotherapy)
- Lymphedema after radiation (experimental at present)
- Anxiety, fright, panic
- Cancer and chemotherapy related tiredness
- Drug detoxification
- Neuralgias

- Certain functional gastro-intestinal disorders (nausea and vomiting after chemotherapy, esophageal spasm, hyperacidity, etc.)
- Headache, migraine, vertigo, tinnitus
- Frozen shoulder
- Cervical and lumbar spine syndromes
- Insomnia
- Anorexia
- Persistent hiccups
- Constipation

Acupuncture performed by professionally qualified practitioners is generally very safe and has very few side effects. The most common side effect is minor bleeding and bruising, which occurs in up to 3% of patients. An acupuncture qualified practitioner specialist can be found in the American Academy of Acupuncture web site. (http://www.medicalacupuncture.org/Find-an-Acupuncturist)

Symptoms and signs of new or recurring head and neck cancer

Most individuals with head and neck cancer receive medical and surgical treatment that removes and eradicates the cancer. However, there is always the possibility that the cancer may recur; vigilance is needed to detect recurrence or possibly new primary tumors. It is therefore important to be aware of the signs of laryngeal and other types of head and neck cancer so that they can be detected at an early stage.

Signs and symptoms of head and neck cancer include:

- Bloody Sputum
- Bleeding from the nose, throat, and mouth
- Lumps on or outside the neck
- Lumps or white, red or dark patches inside the mouth
- Abnormal-sounding or difficult breathing
- Chronic cough
- Changes in one's voice (including hoarseness)
- Neck pain or swelling
- Difficulty chewing, swallowing or moving the tongue
- Thickening of the cheek(s)
- Pain around the teeth, or loosening of the teeth
- A sore in the mouth that doesn't heal or increases in size
- Numbness of the tongue or elsewhere in the mouth
- Persistent mouth, throat or ear pain
- Bad breath
- Weight loss

Individuals with these symptoms should be examined by their otolaryngologists as soon as possible.

Head and neck cancer spread

Head and neck cancers (including laryngeal cancer) can spread to the lungs and the liver. The risk of spread is higher in larger tumors and in tumors that had been recognized late. The greater risk of spread is in the first five years and especially in the first two years after the cancer appears. If local lymph glands have not revealed cancer the risk is lower.

Individuals who had cancer before, may be more likely to develop another type of malignancy not related to their head and neck cancer. As people age they often develop other medical problems that require care, for example, hypertension and diabetes. It is therefore imperative to receive adequate nutrition, take care of one's dental, physical and mental health, be under good medical care and be examined on a regular basis. Head and neck cancer survivors, like everyone else, need to watch for all types of cancers. Some are relatively easy to diagnose by regular examination and include breast, cervix, prostate, colon, and skin cancer.

Low thyroid hormone (hypothyroidism) and its treatment

Most laryngectomees develop low levels of the thyroid hormone (hypothyroidism). This is due to the effects of radiation and/or the removal of part or all of the thyroid gland during laryngectomy surgery.

The symptoms of hypothyroidism vary; some individuals have no symptoms while others have dramatic or, rarely, life-threatening symptoms. The symptoms of hypothyroidism are nonspecific and mimic many normal changes of aging.

General symptoms-The thyroid hormone stimulates the body's metabolism. Most symptoms of hypothyroidism are due to the slowing of metabolic processes. Systemic symptoms include fatigue, sluggishness, feeling down, depressed, weight gain, and intolerance to cold temperatures.

Skin-Decreased sweating, dry and thick skin, coarse or thin hair, disappearance of eyebrows, and brittle nails.

Eyes-Mild swelling around the eyes.

Cardiovascular system-Slowing of the heart rate and weakening of contractions, decreasing its overall function. These can cause fatigue and shortness of breath with exercise. Hypothyroidism can also cause mild hypertension and raise cholesterol levels.

Respiratory system-Respiratory muscles can weaken and lung function can decrease. Symptoms include fatigue, shortness of breath with exercise, and decreased ability to exercise. Hypothyroidism may lead to swelling of the tongue, hoarse voice, and sleep apnea (not in laryngectomees).

Gastrointestinal system-Slowing of the digestive tract motility, causing constipation.

Reproductive system-Menstrual cycle irregularities, ranging from absent or infrequent periods to very frequent and heavy periods.

Thyroid deficiency can be corrected by taking synthetic thyroid hormone (Thyroxine). This should be taken on an empty stomach with a full glass of water 30 minutes before eating, preferably before breakfast or at a similar time of day. This is because food containing high fat (e.g., eggs, bacon, toast, hash brown potatoes, and milk) can decrease thyroxine absorption by 40 percent.

After starting therapy, the patient should be reevaluated and serum thyroid stimulating hormone (TSH) should be measured in three to six weeks, and the dose adjusted if needed. Symptoms of hypothyroidism generally begin to resolve after two to three weeks of replacement therapy and may take at least six weeks to dissipate.

A thyroxine dose can be increased in three weeks in those who continue to have symptoms and who have a high serum TSH concentration. It takes about six weeks before a steady hormone state is achieved after therapy is initiated or the dose is changed.

This process of increasing the dose of hormone every three to six weeks is continued, based upon periodic measurements of TSH until it returns to normal (from approximately 0.5 to 5.0 mU/L). Once this is achieved, periodic monitoring is needed.

After identification of the proper maintenance dose, the patient should be examined and serum TSH measured once a year (or more often if there is an abnormal result or a change in the patient's condition). Dose adjustment may be needed as patients age or have a weight change.

Several formulations of synthetic thyroxine are available, but there has been considerable controversy if they are similar in efficacy. In 2004, the US FDA approved a generic substitute for branded levothyroxine products. The American Thyroid Association, Endocrine Society, and the American Association of Clinical Endocrinologists objected to this decision, recommending that patients remain on the same brand. If patients must switch brands or use a generic substitute, serum TSH should be checked six weeks later.

Because there may be subtle differences between synthetic thyroxine formulations, it is better to stay with one formulation when possible. If the preparation must be changed, follow-up monitoring of TSH and sometimes throxine (T4) serum levels should be done to determine if dose adjustments are necessary.

Lightheadedness, and dizziness

Laryngectomees can experience lightheadedness, and dizziness. It is often due to either side effects of radiation treatment and/or not inhaling enough air when speaking using trachea-esophageal voice prosthesis.

Radiation of the head and neck can damage the peripheral and autonomic nervous system. Dizziness usually occurs when standing up from sitting or lying position due to the development of low blood pressure (orthostatic or postural hypotension). This can be prevented by standing up slowly, wearing compression stockings, exercises and by keeping well hydrated. It is best to consult one's physician to prevent and treat this condition.

Not inhaling enough air while speaking can deprive the brain of oxygen that causes dizziness and lightheadedness. Learning how to speak correctly with the assistance and guidance of a speech and language pathologist can prevent dizziness and lightheadedness.

Speech can be made easier and not lead to lightheadedness and dizziness when following these steps:

- Speaking slowly
- Taking breaks between sentences
- Taking breathes with the stoma not covered
- Speaking slowly
- Speaking only 4-5 words between each air exhalation
- Using diaphragmatic breathing
- Over articulating the words
- Speaking by using low air pressure (in voice prosthesis users)

Constipation

Constipation is common in laryngectomees. This is mainly because they have difficulty in straining in order to have a natural bowel movement. Normally straining is done by closing the vocal cords and increasing the pressure in one's chest by exhaling against the closed vocal cords. The same thing happens when one strain to lift a heavy object. Without a larynx one can't strain normally because the stoma does not allow a laryngectomee to restrict the outflow of air from their lungs. However, some straining is possible after occluding the stoma in those without a voice prosthesis. The straining is less effective in those with a voice prosthesis because some of the exhaled air goes through the voice prosthesis.

What may also contribute to the development of constipation is that laryngectomees may consume less vegetables and fruits because of their swallowing difficulties.

Constipation can be prevented by:

- Consuming a diet that will generate bulk and are high in fiber (fruits, vegetables and grain products) thus reducing dependency on laxatives
- Staying well hydrated by drinking plenty of fluids
- Defecating after meals, taking advantage of normal increases in colonic motility after eating especially in the morning
- Taking a laxative. These include oral bulk forming laxatives (i.e., psyllium or Metamucil, methylcellulose or Citrucel); osmotic agents (polyethylene glycol or Miralax), poorly absorbed or nonabsorbable sugar laxatives (i.e., lactulose , sorbitol), saline laxatives (i.e., Magnesium citrate); and oral (e.g., Dulcolax, Senokot) and rectal stimulant laxatives (e.g., Dulcolax, bisacodyl).
- If possible avoiding medications that cause constipation (i.e., codeine, calcium and iron supplements)
- Reduce consumption of constipation food (i.e., chocolate, bananas, rice)
- Keep active and exercise regularly

Severe constipation can be treated with glycerin suppositories, enema, and by prescribed medications.

Medical and psychological conditions can also induce constipation. These include: hypothyroidism, neuropathy, diabetes, irritable bowel syndrome, and depression. Some medications can also cause constipation. These include: antihistamines, antidepressants, antispasmodics, pain medications (opiates such as codeine), antihypertensives, antacids and calcium and iron supplements.

It is advisable that one seeks medical evaluation and treatment by a physician for their constipation.

Gastroesophageal acid reflux

Most laryngectomees are prone or develop gastroesophageal reflux disease (GERD). (Picture 16) There are two muscular bands or sphincters in the esophagus that prevent reflux. One is located where the esophagus enters the stomach and the other is behind the larynx at the beginning of the esophagus in the neck. The lower esophageal sphincter often becomes compromised when there is a hiatal hernia which may occur in more than 3/4 of people over 70. During laryngectomy the sphincter in the upper esophageal sphincter (the cricopharyngeus) which normally prevents food from returning to the mouth is removed. This leaves the upper part of the esophagus flaccid and always open which may result in the reflux of stomach contents up into the throat and mouth. Therefore, regurgitation of stomach acid and food, especially in the first hour or so after eating, can occur when bending forward or lying down. This can also occur after forceful exhalation when those who use a TEP try to speak.

Taking medications that reduce stomach acidity, such as antacids and proton pump inhibitors (PPI), can alleviate some of the side effects of reflux, such as throat irritation, damage to the gums and bad taste. Not lying down after eating or drinking also helps prevent reflux. Eating small amounts of food multiple times causes less food reflux than eating large meals.

Acid reflux occurs when the acid that is normally in the stomach backs up into the esophagus. This condition is also called GERD.

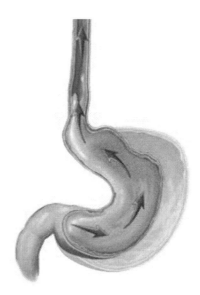

Picture 16: Food reflux from the stomach to the esophagus

Symptoms and treatment of gastroesophageal acid reflux include:

•   Burning in the chest (heartburn)

•   Burning or acid taste in the throat

•   Stomach or chest pain

•   Difficulty in swallowing

•   A raspy voice or a sore throat

•   Unexplained cough (not in laryngectomees, unless their voice prosthesis leaks)

•   In laryngectomees: granulation tissue forms around the voice prosthesis, voice prosthesis device life is shortened, voice problems

Measures that reduce and prevent gastroesophageal acid reflux include:

•   Losing weight (in those who are overweight)

- Reducing stress and practicing relaxation techniques

- Avoiding foods that worsen symptoms (e.g., coffee, chocolate, alcohol, peppermint, and fatty foods)

- Stopping smoking and passive exposure to smoke

- Eating small amounts of food several times a day rather than large meals

- Siting when eating and staying upright 30-60 minutes later

- Avoiding lying down for 2-3 hours after a meal

- Elevating the beds' head side by 6-8 inches (by putting blocks of wood under 2 legs of the bed or a wedge under the mattress) or by using pillows to elevate the upper portion of the body by at least about 45 degrees

- Taking a medication that reduces the production of stomach acids, as prescribed by one's physician

- When bending down, bending the knees rather than bending the upper body

Medications for the treatment of gastroesophageal acid reflux:

There are three major types of medication that can help reduce acid reflux symptoms: antacids, histamine H2-receptor antagonists (also known as H2 blockers), and proton pump inhibitors. These drug classes work in different ways by reducing or blocking stomach acid.

Liquid antacids are generally more active than tablets, and are generally more active if taken after a meal or before going to bed, but they work only for a short time. H2 blockers (e.g., Pepcid, Tagamet, Zantac) work by reducing the amount of acid produced by the stomach. They last longer than antacids and can relieve mild symptoms. Most H2 blockers can be bought without a prescription.

Proton pump inhibitors (e.g., Prilosec, Nexium, Prevacid, Aciphex) are the most effective medicines in treating GERD and stopping the production of stomach acid. Some of these medicines are sold without a prescription. They may reduce the absorption of calcium.

Monitoring the serum calcium levels is important; individuals taking these agents and those with low calcium levels may need to take calcium supplements.

It is advisable to see a physician if the GERD symptoms are severe or last a long time and are difficult to control.

Prevention of medical and surgical errors

Medical and surgical mistakes are very common and are the third leading cause of death in the US leading to 400,000 death a year. The best way of preventing errors is for the patient to be his or her own advocate or to have a family member or friend serve as one's advocate.

Medical errors can be reduced by:

- Being informed and not hesitating to challenge and ask for explanations
- Becoming an "expert" in one's medical issues
- Having family or friends remain in the hospital and accompany one in clinic visits
- Getting a second opinion
- Educating your medical provider about one's condition and needs (prior to and after surgery)

The occurrence of errors weakens patients' trust in their medical providers. Admission and acceptance of responsibility by medical providers can bridge the gap between them and the patient and can reestablish lost confidence. When such a dialogue is established, more details about the circumstances leading to the mistake can be learned thus helping to prevent similar errors. Open discussion can assure patients that their medical providers are taking the mater seriously and that steps will be taken to make their hospital stays safer.

Not discussing mistakes with the patient and family increases their anxiety, frustration and anger, thus interfering with their recovery. And of course, such anger may also lead to malpractice suits.

Greater vigilance by the medical community can reduce errors. Obviously medical errors should be prevented as much as humanly possible; ignoring them can only lead to their repetition. Institutional policies should support and encourage healthcare professionals to disclose adverse events. Increased openness and honesty following adverse events can improve provider-patient relationships. There are important preventive steps that can be implemented by every institution and medical office. Educating the patient, their caregivers, and family members about the patients' condition and treatment plan is of utmost importance. Medical professionals can safeguard and prevent mistakes when they see deviations from the planned therapy.

These steps by the medical establishment can prevent errors:

- Implement better and uniform medical training
- Adhere to well established standards of care
- Perform regular records review to detect and correct medical errors
- Employ only well-educated and trained medical staff
- Counsel, reprimand, and educate staff members who make errors and dismiss those who continue to err
- Develop and meticulously follow algorithms (specific sets of instructions for procedures), establish protocols and bedside checklists for all interventions
- Increase supervision and communication among health care providers
- Investigate all errors and take action to prevent them
- Educate and inform the patient and his/her caregivers about the patient's condition and treatment plans
- Have a family member and or friend serve as a patient advocate to ensure the appropriateness of the management
- Respond to patients' and family complaints. Admit responsibility when appropriate, discuss these with the family and staff and take action to prevent the error(s)

Chapter 13:

Preventive care: follow-up, avoiding smoking and alcohol, preventing thrush, and vaccination

Preventive medical and dental care is essential for patients with cancer. Many individuals with cancer including those with head and neck tumors neglect to attend to other important medical problems and focus exclusively on their cancer. Neglecting other medical issues can lead to serious consequences that may influence wellbeing and longevity. It is important to remember as everyone else, cancer survivors are also susceptible to other ailments. This includes other types of gender and age related cancers (i.e., colon, prostate, breast, skin, etc.)

The most important preventive measures for laryngectomees and other head and neck cancer patients include:

- Proper dental and oral care
- Routine examinations by family physician
- Routine follow-up by an otolaryngologist
- Getting appropriate vaccinations
- Not smoking
- Using proper techniques for caring of airways (e.g., using sterile saline for stoma irrigation)
- Maintaining adequate nutrition

Using proper techniques for stoma care is discussed in **Chapter 8 (page 123)**.

Adequate nutrition is discussed in **Chapter 11 (page 161)**.

Routine dental follow up and dental preventive care are discussed in **Chapter 14 (page 205)**.

Follow-up by family physician, internist and medical specialists

Continual medical follow-up by specialists, including the otolaryngologist, radiation oncologist (for those who received radiation treatment), and oncologist (for those who received chemotherapy), is very important. As time passes after the initial diagnosis and surgery, follow-up occurs with less frequency. Most otolaryngologists recommend monthly follow-up examinations in the first year after diagnosis, and less often afterwards, depending on the patient's condition. Patients should be encouraged to contact their physician whenever new symptoms arise.

Most major cancer medical centers in the US follow the National Comprehensive Cancer Network (NCCN) guidelines and recommendations (https://www.nccn.org/professionals/physician_gls/f_guidelines.asp#site) for follow up of head and neck cancer patients. These guidelines are based on the potential risk of relapse and second primary cancers, treatment sequelae and toxicities to treatment.

They recommend a complete head and neck examination every 1-3 months for the first year after treatment and/or surgery, every 2-6 months for the 2nd year, every 4-8 months for the 3rd through 5th year, and then every 12 months after the fifth year. However, each patient's head and neck surgeon, medical oncologist and/or radiation oncologist generally determines the frequency of follow-up visits based on the relative risk of recurrence, which depends on the site of the original tumor, the stage of the disease when first detected, and whether there was spread of the disease to lymph nodes in the neck or other organs in the body.

They also recommend baseline imaging of the tumor site and also the neck if it has been treated within 6 months of treatment, with further re-imaging as needed based on concerning signs/symptoms, smoking history and areas that can't be seen on a clinical examination. Chest imaging is recommended for individuals with a smoking history based on the guidelines for lung cancer screening. They also recommend a thyroid checkup if the neck has been irradiated or the thyroid has been removed, smoking cessation and alcohol counseling if needed, dental evaluation, a nutritional evaluation and treatment until nutritional status is stabilized, speech/hearing evaluation and swallowing evaluation if needed, and ongoing surveillance for depression.

It is critical that one continues to be vigilant to find out if the cancer returns or if a secondary cancer has emerged. There is a higher probability of cancer returning (recurrence) or a new cancer occurring in the first few years after diagnosis. Early identification of recurrence increases survival; survival is 90% when the cancer is in stage I, and only 70% in stage ll.

It is recommended to undergo periodic follow-up physical examination, scans and other tests according to a schedule. The individual follow-up schedule depends on the cancer's specific type, and the course of treatment given.

Regular checkups ensure that any changes in health are noted and whenever a new problem emerges it is addressed and treated. The clinician will perform a careful examination to detect cancer recurrence. Checkups include a general examination of the entire body and specific examination of the neck, throat and stoma. Examination of the upper airways is performed using an endoscope or indirect visualization with a small, long-handled mirror to check for abnormal areas. Radiological and other studies may also be performed as needed.

The general recommendation is to perform fewer positron emission tomography/ computed tomography (PET/CT) scans the longer the elapsed time from the surgery that removed the cancer. Generally, PET/CT is performed every three to six months during the first year, then every six months during the second and then yearly throughout life. These recommendations, however, are not based on studies and are merely the opinion or consensus among the specialists. More scans are performed if there are concerns or suspicious findings. When scheduling a PET and/or CT scan any potential benefit gained by the information should be weighed against any potential deleterious effects of exposure to ionizing radiation and or X rays.

it is very important to be followed by an internist or family physician, as well as a dentist, to address other medical and dental issues.

Avoiding smoking and alcohol

Smoking and/or excessive alcohol consumption are known risk factors for developing many types of head and neck cancer in addition to several other types of cancer in the body. Individuals with head and neck cancer should receive counseling about the importance of smoking cessation. In addition to being a major risk factor for head and neck cancer, alcohol consumption further enhances the risk of cancer. Smoking can also influence cancer prognosis. Patients with laryngeal cancer who continue to smoke and drink are less likely to be cured and are more likely to develop a second tumor. Continued smoking, either during or after RT, can increase the severity and duration of mucosal reactions, worsen dry mouth (xerostomia), and compromise patient outcome.

Smoking tobacco and drinking alcohol decrease the effectiveness of treatment for laryngeal cancer. Patients who continue to smoke while receiving RD have a lower long-term survival rate than those who do not smoke.

Counseling services are available to help one stop smoking and/or alcohol consumption. There also are medications approved by the United States Food and Drug Administration (FDA) that can help stop smoking.

Preventing thrush

Thrush can occur as a result of radiation treatment, chemotherapy, high carbohydrate intake, antibiotic or steroid treatment, and poor oral hygiene. Oral thrush (also called oral candidiasis) is caused by the fungus *Candida albicans*. Candida is a normal inhabitant of the mouth that can overgrow and cause clinical symptoms such as thrush. Oral thrush causes creamy white lesions, usually on the tongue or inner cheeks. Sometimes oral thrush may spread to the roof of the mouth, gums, tonsils, and the back of the throat. Undergoing chemotherapy and/or radiation treatment, and having conditions that lead to a dry mouth predisposes to thrush.

One's physician may recommend antifungal medication(s). These comes in several forms, including lozenges, tablets, or a liquid that one can swish in their mouth and then swallow.

There are several methods that help prevent yeast growth in the mouth:

- Reduce the consumption of sugars in food and drinks, brush your teeth well after consuming sugary food and/or drinks
- Brush your teeth well after every meal and especially before going to sleep.
- Diabetic should maintain adequate blood sugar levels
- Take antibiotics or corticosteroids only if they are needed
- If one uses an oral suspension of an antifungal agent, one should wait for 30 minutes to let it work and then brush your teeth. This is because some of these suspensions contain sugar
- Consume probiotics by eating active-culture yogurt and/or a probiotic preparation
- Gently brush the tongue if it is coated with yeast (white plaques). Brushing should be avoided in those who have irradiation mucositis
- Replace the toothbrush after overcoming a yeast problem to prevent re colonization with yeasts

Vaccinations

Vaccination is the most cost effective way by which infections can be prevented. It can protect the vaccinated person as well as those around them from becoming infected; reduce the need for antibiotics and antiviral agents; prevent hospitalizations and prolong life.

Laryngectomees are directly exposed to airborne respiratory pathogens (i.e., viruses, bacteria) because the air they inhale is no longer filtered by the nasal mucosa. This makes them more susceptible to lower respiratory tract and other infections that access the body through the respiratory tract. This is why it is very important to get vaccinated against all respiratory tract pathogens.

It is important for laryngectomees to be vaccinated for respiratory infections caused by viruses (e.g., influenza) and bacteria (e.g., *Streptococcus pneumoniae*) and shingles (herpes zoster virus). Preventing or reducing the severity of these infections is recommended by the Center of Disease Control and Prevention (CDC).

Influenza (flu) vaccination: It is important for laryngectomees to be vaccinated for influenza regardless of age. Influenza can be more difficult to manage and vaccination is an important preventive tool.

There are two types of influenza vaccine: an injection that is adequate for all ages and an inhalation (live virus) only given to individuals younger than 50 years who are not immuno-compromised.

A new vaccine for influenza is prepared for every new winter season. While the exact strains that cause influenza are unpredictable, it is likely that strains that caused the illness at other parts of the world will also cause illness in the U.S. It is best to consult one's physician prior to vaccination to ensure that there is no reason why one should not be vaccinated (such as egg allergy).

How well the flu vaccine prevents flu varies from season to season. The vaccine's effectiveness also can vary depending on who is being vaccinated. At least two factors play an important role in determining the likelihood that flu vaccine will protect a person from flu illness: 1) characteristics of the person being vaccinated (i.e., their age and health), and 2) the similarity or "match" between the flu viruses the flu vaccine is designed to protect against and the flu viruses spreading in the community. During years when the flu vaccine is not well matched to circulating viruses, it's possible that no or only little benefit from flu vaccination may be observed.

The best way to diagnose Influenza is a rapid test of nasal secretions by one of the diagnostic kits. Because laryngectomees have no connection between the nose and the lungs, it is advisable to test nasal secretions in addition to tracheal sputum (using a kit that was approved for sputum testing).

Information about these recommendation for vaccination and diagnostic tests can be found in the Center of Disease Control website. https://www.cdc.gov/flu/

One "advantage" of being a laryngecomee is that one generally gets fewer infections caused by respiratory tract viruses. This is because "cold" viruses generally first infect the nose and throat; from there they travel to the rest of the body, including the lungs. Because laryngectomees do not breathe through their nose; cold viruses are less likely to infect them.

It is still important for laryngectomees to receive yearly immunization for influenza viruses, to wear a Heat and Moisture Exchanger (HME) device to filter the air that gets into the lungs, and to wash their hands well before touching the stoma or the HME, or before eating. The Atos (Provox) Micron HME with electrostatic filter is designed to filtrate potential pathogens and to reduce susceptibility to respiratory infections.

The influenza virus is capable of spreading by touching objects. Laryngectomees who use a voice prosthesis and need to press their HME to speak may be at increased risk of introducing the virus directly to their lungs. Washing hands or using a skin cleanser can prevent the spread of the virus.

Vaccination against the pneumococcal bacteria: It is advisable that laryngectomees and other neck breathers get vaccinated against the pneumococcus bacterium (*Streptococcus pneumoniae*) which is one of the major causes of pneumonia. In the United States there are two types of vaccines against the pneumococcal bacteria: the pneumococcal conjugate vaccine (Prevnar 13 or PCV13) and the pneumococcal polysaccharaide vaccine-a 23-valent pneumococcal polysaccharide vaccine (Pneumovax or PPV23).

One should consult their physician about receiving the pneumococcal vaccination.

The Center for Disease Control publishes the current vaccination guidelines at:

https://www.cdc.gov/vaccines/vpd/pneumo/hcp/index.html

Vaccination for *Haemophilus influenzae* Type b (Hib): Hib vaccine prevents serious infections caused by a bacteria called Haemophilus influenzae type b. Such infections include meningitis, pneumonia, and epiglottitis. Children older than five years and adults usually do not need Hib vaccine. But it may be recommended for older children or adults with no spleen or sickle cell disease, or following a bone marrow transplant. Because of the increased risk of laryngectomees to be infected with respiratory tract pathogens the administration of this vaccine may be considered.

The Center for Disease Control publishes the current vaccination guidelines are:

https://www.cdc.gov/vaccines/hcp/vis/vis-statements/hib.html

Vaccination for Neisseria meningitides: Meningococcal Disease is a type of illness caused by *Neisseria meningitidis* bacteria. There are three types of meningococcal vaccines. There are two types of meningococcal vaccines available in the United States: Meningococcal conjugate vaccines and Serogroup B meningococcal vaccines. The CDC recommends that all 11 to 12 year olds should be vaccinated with a meningococcal conjugate vaccine. A booster dose is recommended at age 16 years. Teens and young adults (16 through 23 year olds) also may be vaccinated with a serogroup B meningococcal vaccine. In certain situations, other children and adults could be recommended to get meningococcal vaccines. Because of the increased risk of laryngectomees to be infected with respiratory tract pathogens the administration of this vaccine may be considered.

The Center for Disease Control publishes the current vaccination guidelines are:

https://www.cdc.gov/vaccines/vpd/mening/index.html

Vaccination for shingles (Herpes zoster): Shingles (Herpes zoster) is a painful skin rash caused by the varicella (chicken post) zoster virus. Shingles usually appears in a band, a strip, or a small area on one side of the face or body.

Shingles is most common in older adults and people with weak immune system because of stress, injury, certain medicines, or other reasons. Vaccine for shingles (Zostavax®) is recommended by the CDC for people older than 60 years to prevent shingles and reduce pain after the infection in those who still get shingles. The vaccine reduced the risk of getting shingles by about half and the risk of pain along a nerve (neuralgia) in those that who still get shingle by 2/3. The older a person is, the more severe the effects of shingles typically are, so all adults older than 60 years should get vaccinated regardless of whether they had chickenpox or not.

The shingles vaccine is not recommended to treat active shingles or post-herpetic neuralgia (pain after the rash is gone) once it develops. It should not be administered to those allergic to gelatin, neomycin, or any components of shingles vaccine; those with a weakened immune system (i.e., HIV/AIDS, leukemia, lymphoma, steroids, receiving radiation or chemotherapy); and those who are pregnant. One should check with their physician to make sure they can be vaccinated.

In 2017 the US Food and Drug Administration approved a second shingles vaccine (Shingrix®) that offered greater protection than the previous vaccine. It consists of a lyophilized recombinant varicella zoster virus (VZV) glycoprotein E antigen combined with an adjuvant that enhances its efficacy.

Chapter 14:

Dental Issues and hyperbaric oxygen therapy

Dental issues can be challenging for laryngectomees, mainly because of the long term effects of RD. Maintenance of good dental hygiene can prevent many problems.

Dental Issues

Dental problems are common after exposure of the head and neck to RD.

Long term effects of radiation on the oral cavity include:

- Reduced blood supply to the maxillary and mandibular bones.
- Reduced production and changes in the chemical composition of saliva.
- Changes in the bacteria that colonize the mouth.

Because of these effects dental caries, soreness, and gingival and periodontal inflammation can be particularly problematic. These can be lessened by maintaining good oral and dental hygiene that include cleaning, flossing, and use of fluoridated toothpaste after each meal when possible. Using a special fluoridated preparation to gargle or apply on the gum helps in preventing dental carries. Keeping well hydrated and using saliva substitute when needed are also important.

It is advisable that patients receiving RD to the head and neck visit their dentist for a thorough oral examination several weeks prior to initiation of the treatment and be examined at a regular semiannual or annual basis throughout life. Getting regular dental cleaning by a dental hygienist or a dentist are also important.

Because radiation treatment alters the blood supply to the maxillary and mandibular bones patients may be at risk of developing bone necrosis (osteoradionecrosis) at those sites. Tooth extraction, dental implants and dental disease in irradiated areas can lead to the development of osteoradionecrosis. Patients should inform their dentist about their past radiation treatment prior to these procedures. The risk of developing osteoradionecrosis may be reduced by administration of a series of hyperbaric oxygen therapy (see below) before and after extraction or dental surgery. This is recommended if the involved teeth, or planned implants are at an area that had been exposed to a high dose of radiation. Consulting the radiation oncologist who delivered the radiation treatment can be helpful in determining if this is necessary.

Dental prophylaxis can reduce the risk of developing dental problems leading to bone necrosis. Special fluoride treatments may help to prevent dental problems, along with brushing, flossing, and having one's teeth cleaned regularly.

A home care dental lifelong routine is recommended:

- Flossing each tooth and brushing with toothpaste after each meal.
- Brushing the tongue with a tongue brush or a soft bristled toothbrush once a day.
- Rinsing with a baking soda rinse daily. Baking soda helps neutralize the mouth. The rinse is made of one teaspoon of baking soda added to 12 oz. of water. The baking soda rinse can be used throughout the day.
- Using fluoride in a fluoride tray once a day. These preparation are commercially available and are can also be custom made by dentists. They are applied over the teeth for 10 minutes. One should not rinse, drink, or eat for 30 minutes after fluoride application.

Gastroesophageal acid reflux is also very common after head and neck surgery, especially in individuals who have had partial or complete laryngectomy. (see **Gastroesophageal reflux, Chapter 12, page 191**) This can also cause dental erosion (especially of the lower jaw) and, ultimately teeth loss. Measures to reduce and prevent acid reflux can be found in **Chapter 11, page 192)**.

Hyperbaric oxygen therapy

Hyperbaric oxygen (HBO) therapy involves breathing pure oxygen in a pressurized room. HBO is a well-established treatment for decompression sickness (a hazard of scuba diving) and can be used to prevent osteoradionecrosis.

HBO is used to treat a wide range of medical conditions including: bubbles of air in the blood vessels (arterial gas embolism), decompression sickness, carbon monoxide poisoning, a wound that won't heal, a crush injury, gangrene, skin or bone infection causing tissue death (such as osteoradionecrosis; **page 58**), radiation injuries, burns, skin grafts or skin flaps at risk of tissue death, and severe anemia.

HBO therapy alone can often effectively treat decompression sickness, arterial gas embolism and severe carbon monoxide poisoning. To effectively treat other conditions, HBO therapy is used as part of a comprehensive treatment plan and is administered in conjunction with additional therapies and medications that fit individual needs.

To be effective, HBO therapy requires more than one session. The number of sessions required depends on the medical condition. Some conditions, such as carbon monoxide poisoning, can be treated in as few as three visits. Others, such as osteoradionecrosis, and non-healing wounds, may require 20 to 30 treatments. Those who require dental extraction are often 20 treatments prior to the procedure and 10 following it.

HBO can be used in patients with head and neck cancer for the treatment of osteoradionecrosis, refractory osteomyelitis, dental procedures (i.e., extractions), avert the risk of flap or graft failure, and necrotizing soft tissue and wound infections. Antibiotics are administered in conjunction with HBO to those with infections.

In an HBO therapy chamber, the air pressure is raised up to three times higher than normal air pressure. Under these conditions, the lungs can gather much more oxygen than would be possible when breathing pure oxygen at normal air pressure.

The blood carries this oxygen throughout the body, stimulating the release of chemicals called "growth factors" and stem cells that promote healing. When tissue is injured, it requires even more oxygen to survive. HBO therapy increases the amount of oxygen in the blood and can temporarily restore normal levels of blood gases and tissue function. These promote healing and the ability of the tissues to fight infection.

There is no evidence indicating that HBO neither acts as a stimulator of tumor growth nor as an enhancer of recurrence. On the other hand, there is evidence that implies that HBO might have tumor-inhibitory effects in certain cancer subtypes.

HBO therapy can be performed as outpatient procedure and does not require hospitalization. Hospitalized patients may need to be transported to and from the HBO therapy site if it is an outside facility.

Treatment can be performed in one of two settings:

- A unit designed for one person in an individual (monoplace) unit where the patient lies down on a padded table that slides into a clear plastic tube.
- A chamber designed to accommodate several people in a multiperson HBO room where the patient may sit or lie down. A hood or mask delivers the oxygen.

During HBO therapy the increased air pressure creates a temporary feeling of fullness in the ears-similar to the one felt in an airplane or at a high altitude that can be relieved by yawning.

A therapy session may last from one to two hours. Members of the health care team monitor the patient throughout the session. Following HBO therapy the patient may feel lightheaded. Typically, this feeling dissipates within a few minutes.

HBO is relatively safe and complications are rare. Most complications are caused by the increased air pressure and volume barotrauma in the middle ear (i.e., tympanic membrane rupture), sinuses, and lungs. Other complication include increased heart output, seizure activity as a result of oxygen toxicity, and effects on the eye (i.e., temporary nearsightedness or myopia, and enhancing a cataract).

HBO is absolutely contraindicated in those with untreated pneumothorax. It is relatively contraindicated in those with claustrophobia (who can be pretreated with anti-anxiety medications), advanced congestive heart failure or obstructive lung disease, bullous lung disease, while receiving chemotherapy, seizure disorder, active smoking, pregnancy, chronic sinus congestion, and fever.

Pure oxygen can cause a fire if there is a source of ignition, such as a spark or flame, and adequate fuel. It is therefore forbidden to take items that could ignite a fire (e.g., lighters or battery powered devices) into the HBO therapy room.

The risk of fire inside the chamber can be averted by with these safety measures:

- Patients should wear cotton cloth and gown
- Avoiding the use of battery operated devices inside the chamber. Medical devices (i.e., pacemaker, defibrillator) are allowed after they have been tested.
- Avoiding cosmetics
- No newspaper, tobacco products or matches are allowed
- Grounding the patient with a wire

Chapter 15:

Psychological issues: depression, suicide, uncertainty, disfigurement, PTSD, sharing the diagnosis, and source of support in head and neck cancer patients

Head and neck cancer survivors, including laryngectomees, face many psychological, social and personal challenges. This is mainly because head and neck cancer and its treatment affect some of the most basic human functions-breathing, eating, communication, and social interaction. Understanding and treating these issues are no less important than dealing with medical concerns. Post-traumatic stress disorder (see below) is one of the psychological results of laryngectomy and is more common in females.

Individuals diagnosed with cancer experience numerous feelings and emotions which can change from day to day, hour to hour, or even minute to minute and can generate a heavy psychological burden.

Some of the feelings are: denial, anger, mood swings, fear, stress, anxiety, depression, sadness, guilt, and loneliness.

Some of the psychological and social challenges faced by laryngectomees include: depression; anxiety and fear of recurrence; social isolation; substance abuse; body image; sexuality, return to work; interaction with spouse, family, friends, and co-workers; and economic impact.

Coping with depression

Many people with cancer feel sad or depressed. This is a normal response to any serious illness. Depression is one of the most difficult issues faced by a patient with cancer. Yet the social stigma associated with admitting depression makes it difficult to reach out and seek therapy.

Some of the signs of depression include:

- A feeling of helplessness and hopelessness, or that life has no meaning
- No interest in being with family or friends
- Inability to communicate
- Difficulty paying attention
- No interest in the hobbies and activities one used to enjoy
- A loss of appetite, or no interest in food
- Crying for long periods of time, or many times each day
- Sleep problems, either sleeping too much or too little
- Changes in energy level and apathy
- Wide mood swings raging from elation to despair
- Feeling isolated
- Changes in sexual desire
- Thoughts of suicide, including making plans or taking action to kill oneself, as well as frequently thinking about death and dying.

The challenges of life as a laryngectomee in the shadow of cancer means that it is even more difficult to deal with depression. Being unable to speak, or even having difficulties with speaking, make it harder to express emotions and can lead to isolation. Surgical and medical care is often not sufficient to address such issues; more emphasis should be given to mental well-being after laryngectomy.

Coping with and overcoming depression are very important, not only for the well-being of the patient, but also may facilitate recovery, and increase one's chance for longer survival and ultimate cure. There is growing scientific evidence of a connection between mind and body. Although many of these connections are not yet understood, it is well recognized that individuals who are motivated to get better and exhibit a positive attitude recover faster from serious illnesses, live longer and sometimes survive immense odds. Indeed, it has been shown that this effect may be mediated by alterations in the cellular immune responses and a decrease in natural killer cell activity.

There are, of course many reasons to feel depressed after learning one's cancer diagnosis and, then, living with it. It is a devastating illness for patients and their families, even more so because medicine has not yet found a cure for most types of cancer. By the time the disease has been discovered, it is too late for prevention and, if the cancer has been discovered at an advanced stage, the risk of dissemination is high and the chance of ultimate cure significantly decreased.

Many emotions run through the patient's mind after learning the bad news. "Why me?" and "Can it be true?" Depression is part of the normal mechanism of coping with adversity. Most people go through several stages in coping with a difficult new situation such as becoming a laryngectomee. At first one undergoes denial and isolation, than anger, followed by depression, and finally acceptance.

Some people get "stuck" at a certain stage, such as depression or anger. It is important to move on and get to the final stage of acceptance and eventually hope. This is why professional help as well as understanding and help, by family and friends are important.

Patients have to face their ultimate mortality, sometimes for the first time in their lives. They are forced to deal with the illness and its immediate and long term consequences. Paradoxically, feeling depressed after learning about the diagnosis allows the patient to accept the new reality. Not caring any more makes it easier to live with an uncertain future. While thinking that "I do not care anymore " may make it temporary easier for a while, such a coping mechanism may interfere with seeking appropriate care and can lead to a rapid decline in one's quality of life.

Overcoming depression

Hopefully a patient can find the strength within to fight depression. Immediately after a laryngectomy individuals may be overwhelmed by new daily tasks and realities. They often experience a mourning period for their many losses, which include their voice and their prim state of health. They also have to accept many permanent deficits including not being able to speak "normally". Some may feel that they have a choice between succumbing to a creeping depression or becoming proactive and returning to life. A desire to get better and overcome a handicap can be the driving force to reversing the downhill trend. Depression may recur, requiring a continuous struggle to overcome it.

Some of the ways laryngectomee and head and neck cancer patients can overcome depression include:

- Avoid substance abuse
- Seek help from your doctor, nurse, or a member of your health care team with whom you feel comfortable
- Exclude medical causes (e.g., hypothyroidism, side effect of medication)
- Determine to become proactive
- Minimize stress
- Set an example for others
- Return to previous activities
- Talk to a psychologist or social worker
- Consider antidepressant medication
- Seek support from family, friends, professional, colleagues, fellow laryngectomees, and support groups

These are some of the ways of renewing one's spirit:

- Develop leisure activities

- Build personal relationships
- Keep physically fit and active
- Social reintegration with family and friends
- Volunteer
- Find purposeful projects
- Rest

Support by family members and friends is very important. Continuous involvement and contribution to others lives can be invigorating. One can draw strength from enjoying, interacting and impacting the lives of their children and grandchildren. Setting an example to one's children and grandchildren not to give up in the face of adversity can be the driving force to be proactive and resist depression.

Getting involved in activities one liked before the surgery can provider a continuous purpose for life. Participating in the activities of a local laryngectomee club can be a new source of support, advice and friendship.

Seeking the help of a mental health professional such as a social worker, psychologist or psychiatrist can also be very helpful. There are many treatment options available to treat the depression. These include psychotherapy, medications, and transcranial magnetic stimulation. Having a caring and competent physician and a speech and language pathologist who can provide continuous follow-up is very important. Their involvement can help patients deal with emerging medical and speech problems and can contribute to their sense of well-being.

Suicide among head and neck cancer patients

The suicide rate in cancer patients is twice of that of the general population according to recent studies. These studies clearly point to the urgent need to recognize and treat psychiatric problems such as depression and suicidal ideation in patients.

Most studies have found high incidence of depressive mood disorders associated with suicide among cancer patients. In addition to major and minor depressive disorders, there is also a high rate of less severe depression in elderly cancer patients which is sometimes not recognized and often undertreated. Many studies have shown that in about half of all suicides among people with cancer, major depression was present. There are other important contributory factors that include anxiety, lack of social support systems, and demoralization.

Screening cancer patients for depression, hopelessness, distress, severe pain, coping problems, and suicidal ideation is a useful way to identify those at risk. Counseling and referral to mental health specialists when appropriate may prevent suicide in at-risk cancer patients. This approach also involves speaking with patients at heightened risk for suicide (and their families) about reducing their access to the most common methods used to commit suicide.

Coping with uncertain future

Once one has been diagnosed with cancer and even after successful treatment, it is difficult and close to impossible to completely free oneself from the fear that it may return. Some people are better than others in living with this uncertainty; those who adjust well end up being happier and are more able to go on with their lives than those who do not.

One of the difficult challenges is waiting for the results of an important test or scan (i.e., PET or CT). Many individuals feel anxiety and are worried during the waiting period. Hopefully, the results of such tests are made available without a long delay.

What makes predicting the future difficult is that the scans used to detect cancer (positron emission tomography or PET, magnetic resonance imaging or MRI, and computed tomography or CT) only detect cancer that is larger than one centimeter; physicians may miss a small lesion located at a site that is difficult to visualize.

Patients have therefore to accept the reality that the cancer may return and that physical examination and vigilance are the best ways of monitoring their condition.

What often helps with coping with a new symptom (unless it is urgent) is to wait a few days before seeking medical assistance. In general the majority of new symptoms will go away within a short period. Over time, most people learn not to panic and to use past experience, common sense, and their knowledge to rationalize and understand their symptoms.

Hopefully, over time, one gets better in coping with an uncertain future and learns to accept it, and live with it, striking a balance between fear and acceptance.

Some suggestions how to cope with the uncertain future include:

• Separating oneself from the illness

• Focusing on interests other than cancer

• Developing a life style that avoids stress and promotes inner peace

• Continuing with regular medical check-ups

Post-traumatic stress disorder (PTSD) after head and neck surgery

Post-traumatic stress disorder (PTSD) symptoms may start within three months of a traumatic event. This can occur in 24% of patients who survived intensive care unit (ICU) hospitalization, and up to 11% of those undergoing laryngectomy. It is characterized by intrusive thoughts, nightmares and flashbacks of past traumatic events, avoidance of reminders of trauma, hypervigilance, and sleep disturbance. These individuals compensate for such intense arousal by attempting to avoid experiences that may begin to elicit symptoms; this can result in emotional numbing, diminished interest in everyday activities and, in the extreme, may result in detachment from others.

Symptoms include:

Intrusive memories:

- Recurrent, unwanted distressing memories of the traumatic event
- Reliving the traumatic event as if it were happening again (flashbacks)
- Upsetting dreams about the traumatic event
- Severe emotional distress or physical reactions to thing that reminds one of the event

Avoidance:

- Trying to avoid thinking or talking about the traumatic event
- Avoiding places, activities or individuals that remind one of the traumatic event

Negative changes in thinking and mood:

- Negative feelings about oneself or other persons
- Inability to have positive emotions
- Feeling emotionally numbness
- Lack of interest in activities one used to enjoy
- Hopelessness about one's future
- Memory problems, including not remembering everything about the traumatic event
- Difficulty maintaining close relationships

Changes in emotional reactions:

- Irritability, angry outbursts or aggressive behavior
- Always being on guard for danger
- Overwhelming guilt or shame
- Self-destructive behavior, such as overdrinking or risk taking
- Trouble concentrating
- Trouble sleeping
- Being easily startled or frightened

PTSD treatment can help regaining a sense of control over one's life. Psychotherapy is the main treatment, but often includes medication. Combining these treatments can help improve the symptoms, and teach skills to address the symptoms, help one feel better about themselves and learn ways to cope if any symptoms arise again.

Psychotherapeutic treatment of PTSD includes:

- Cognitive therapy helps recognizing the ways of thinking (cognitive patterns) that are keeping one stuck-for example, negative or inaccurate ways of perceiving normal situations.
- Exposure therapy helps safely face what one finds frightening so that one can learn to cope with it effectively.
- Group therapy can also offer a way to connect with others going through similar experiences.

Sharing the diagnosis with others

After being diagnosed with cancer one has to decide whether to share the information with others or keep it private. Individuals may choose to keep the information private out of fear of stigmatization, rejection or discrimination. Some do not want to show vulnerability and weakness or feel that they are pitied by others. Acknowledged or not, sick people-especially those with a potentially terminal illness – are less able to be competitive in society and are often intentionally or unintentionally discriminated against. Some may fear that otherwise compassionate friends and acquaintances may distance themselves in order to be protected from a perceived inevitable loss-or simply because they do not know what to say or how to behave.

Keeping the diagnosis private can create emotional isolation and burdens as one faces the new reality without support. Some may share the diagnosis only with a limited number of people to spare others from the emotional trauma. Of course, asking people to keep this often devastating information private deprives them from receiving their own emotional support and assistance.

Sharing the information with family and friends may be difficult and is best presented in a way that suits the individual's coping abilities. It is best to communicate one on one and to allow each person to ask questions and express their feelings, fears and concerns. Delivering the news in an optimistic fashion, highlights the potential for recovery, can make it easier. Telling young children can be challenging and is best done according to their abilities to digest the information.

Following surgery, and especially after a laryngectomy it is no longer possible to hide the diagnosis. Most people do not regret sharing their diagnosis with others. They generally discover that their friends do not abandon them and they receive support and encouragement which helps them through difficult times. By "getting out of the closet" and sharing their diagnosis, survivors are making a statement that they do not feel ashamed or weak because of their illness.

Laryngectomees are a small group among cancer survivors. Yet they are in a unique position because they bear their diagnoses on their neck and through their voice. They cannot hide the fact that they breathe through their stomas and speak with weak and sometimes mechanical voices. Yet their survivorship is a testament that a productive and meaningful life is possible even after being diagnosed with cancer.

Coping and adjusting to one's disfigurement

Dealing with disfigurement of the face and neck as a result of surgery and radiation is one of the greatest challenges for laryngectomees. It may influence their self-image and self- identity. Cancer and its treatment can cause significant changes to how one looks, feels and functions. For many whose appearance changed significantly after treatment, adjusting to their new looks and/or impaired ability to communicate and/or eat is very difficult.

Unlike many other types of cancer, the deformities and scars from head and neck cancer are often visible and cannot be hidden. This may make one feel self-conscious and less confident than they were before, and may make one wonder if these visible disfigurements will influence their relationships. It may push some to social isolation and depression. However, one can still enjoy a happy and productive life if one learns to accept these changes, and take advantage of the help available and find ways to adapt to their new reality.

Hopefully, over time one can adjust to their disfigurements. These adjustments require dealing with physical, emotional and social issues. Physical adjustments include dealing with difficulties in drinking, chewing, swallowing, breathing, speaking, hearing and head and neck movements. These issues may affect one's social adjustment as they may limit one's ability to eat out or enjoy other social interactions and can lead to isolation. The need to find new ways to communicate can be frustrating and difficult. Overcoming one's functional challenges and fears about how others may react to them is an important step in adjustment. Maintaining an active social life can assist, prevent or reverse depression, anxiety and isolation.

Adjusting to changes in appearance and function can be very challenging. The face and neck are visible and it is there where individuals express their emotions. Many individuals feel self-conscious or even afraid of social interactions because they are uncertain how people will react to them. Even though it is difficult to control how others will react, there are coping strategies that can help one interact more confidently and/or avoid negative encounters. Clinical research showed that individuals with facial disfigurements who approach others with confidence and the belief that they will accept their appearance are more likely to be successful socially and emotionally than those who are not confident or expect rejection. Most people will respond positively and adapt quickly to one's appearance and will react better to those who are confident and positive. A potentially positive and an uplifting consequence of openly displaying their deformities is that this reveals one's medical history and the fact that one is a cancer survivor who goes on with their life despite their handicap.

Sources of social and emotional support

Learning that one has laryngeal or any head and neck cancer can change the individual's life and the lives of those close to them. These changes can be difficult to handle. Seeking help to better cope with the psychological and social impact of the diagnosis is very important.

The emotional burden includes concerns about treatment and its side effects, hospital stays, and the economic impact of the illness including how to deal with medical bills. Additional worries are directed how to interact with one's family, keeping one's work, and continuing one's daily activities.

Reaching out to other laryngectomees and head and neck cancer support groups can be helpful. Hospital and home visits by fellow survivors can provide support and advice and can facilitate recovery. Fellow laryngetomees and head and neck cancer survivors frequently provide guidance and set an example for successful recovery and the ability to return to a full and rewarding life.

Sources for support include:

- Members of the health care team (physicians, nurses, and speech and language pathologists) can answer and clarify questions about treatment, work, or other activities.
- Social workers, counselors, or members of the clergy can be helpful if one wishes to share one's feelings or concerns. Social workers can suggest resources for financial aid, transportation, home care, and emotional support.

- Support groups for laryngectomees and other individuals with head and neck cancer meet with patients and their family members and share what they have learned about coping with cancer. Groups may also offer support in person, over the telephone, or on the Internet. Member of the health care team may be able to help in finding support groups.

A complete list of potential resources can be found at the **Addendum (page 252)**

Some "Benefits" of being a laryngectomee

There are some "benefits" being a laryngectomee.

These are:

- No more snoring
- Excuse not to wear a tie
- Not smelling offensive or irritating odors
- Experiencing fewer colds
- Low risk of aspiration into the lungs
- Easier to intubate through the stoma in an emergency

Chapter 16:

The caregiver's and partner's needs, sexuality and intimacy in head and neck cancer patients

The caregiver's role and needs

Caregiver's needs and emotional burden

Being a caregiver for a loved one with a serious illness such as head and neck cancer is very difficult and can be physically and emotionally taxing. It can be extremely hard to watch the person they care for suffer especially if there is little that they can do to reverse the illness. Caregivers should, however, realize the importance of what they are doing even when they get no or little appreciation.

Caregivers often experience similar emotions and psychological strains as the person they care for. These include fear, anxiety and distress. They may fear the potential death of their loved one and life without them. This can be very anxiety provoking and depressing. Some cope by refusing to accept the diagnosis of cancer and believe that their loved ones illness is less serious in nature.

Caregivers often sacrifice their own well-being and needs to accommodate those of the person they care for. They often have to calm down their loved one's fears and support them despite being often the target of their vented anger, frustrations and anxieties. These frustrations may be exaggerated in those with head and neck cancer who have often difficulties in expressing themselves verbally. Caregivers frequently suppress their own feelings and hide their own emotions so as not to upset the sick person. This is very taxing and difficult.

It is very useful for the patient and their caregivers to openly and honestly talk to each other sharing their feelings, worries, and aspirations. This may be more challenging in those who have difficulties in speaking. Jointly meeting the health care providers allows for better communication and facilitates shared decision making.

Unfortunately, the well-being of caregivers is frequently ignored as all the attention is focused on the sick individual. It is essential, however, that the needs of the caregivers are not ignore. Getting physical and emotional support from friends, family, support groups, and mental health professionals can be very helpful for the caregiver. Professional counseling can be obtained in an individual setting or support group with or without other family members and the patient. They should find time for themselves to "recharge" their own batteries. Having time dedicated to their own needs can help them continue to be a source of support and strength to their loved one.

Places where a caretaker can turn for support include:

- Family members or friends who will listen without judgment
- One's church, temple, or other place of worship
- Caregiver support groups at a local hospital or online
- A therapist, social worker, or counselor
- National caregiver organizations
- Organizations specific to one's family member's illness or disability

The patient's needs

Because treatment of head and neck cancer (radiation, chemotherapy and surgery) induces fatigue the caregiver may need to assume many supportive roles:

- Assist with daily errands and tasks such as shopping, doing chores or providing transportation to medical appointments.

- Help in preparing meals and feed the patient if needed.
- Assist in daily hygiene (taking a bath, washing hands etc.)
- Assist in providing medical care, including administering oral medication.
- Help in managing administrative issues such as medical insurance reimbursement.
- Providing emotional support and assisting in obtaining professional help if needed.
- Accompany the patient to medical appointments and assist in making medical decisions about treatment and testing choices.
- Help in solving problem by exploring options and making decisions.
- Help in childcare responsibilities.

The caregiver's assistance plays a major and invaluable role in the patient's recovery and recuperation.

The impact of a laryngectomy on the patient's spouse or partner

Many clinicians focused only on the psychosocial impact of head and neck cancer on their patients. However, head and neck cancer has a considerable psychosocial impact on the patient's partner. The partner can experience an even higher psychological stress level than the patients which can hamper adequate care to the patients.

Healthcare professionals should include the partner in the support they offer their patients. The partners of laryngectomees often neglect their own psychosocial problems and consequently cannot provide support for the patient and are at risk of developing medical or psychosocial issues themselves. Healthcare professionals should, therefore, not only implement structural screening and treatment for patients, but also for their partners.

Laryngectomy can effect the patients and partners in a different way. Partners may develop anxiety, fear and concern about the potential death of the laryngectomee and feelings of irritation in social settings. Partners can sometimes become overprotective, which may have a negative impact on their relationship with the laryngectomee. Some partners may be more vulnerable to negative impact of the laryngectomy on their individual psychosocial well-being. These include female partners, those with a lower educational background and older partners.

Discussing the consequences of the laryngectomy with the partner or spouse and the family

It is important to discuss and prepare the patient's spouse or partners as well as family members for the consequences of the laryngectomy. A considerable number of laryngectomees and partners talk as little as possible about the laryngectomy because they do not want to upset others. Openly discussing the illness and its related matters in the family was found to be an important predictor of positive rehabilitation outcomes in head and neck cancer patients. The more open patients are to discuss their experience, the fewer negative feelings such as depression, anxiety and less loss of control are reported. Couples who do not openly discuss the illness should be offered support in order to improve their communication and indirectly improve their quality of life and possibly the quality of their relationship.

There is a substantial group of laryngectomees with feelings of dependency on their partner and that may overburden them. Both patients and partners should be prepared, as a team, by professionals, on the possible changes in their life after a laryngectomy.

The impact of laryngectomy on sexuality and intimacy

The loss of sexuality and intimacy between the laryngectomee and their partner can add a profound burden that is often magnified by the lack of discussion about this topic. Sexuality and intimacy should be addressed in the screening and management of both patients and their partners. The decreased frequency of sexuality, as well as the experience itself need to be dealt with. Issue that may affect sexuality include concern about respiration problems during intercourse, shame related to the stoma and disfigurement and the feeling of not being a complete man or woman anymore. Disfigurement and dysfunction as a result of the cancer and its treatment can cause individuals to feel less attractive. Patients and their partners should be encouraged to discuss issues about sexuality and intimacy. Unfortunately, some clinicians find it difficult to address these topics because of a lack of time, experience and preparation.

The first step in addressing these issues is for the medical professional (physician or nurse) to talk to the patient and their partner about these intimate issues. A trained and experienced professional should listen to the couple, and provide information, advice and psychological support. Based on screening and clinical judgment they may choose to refer the couple to a specialized social worker or psychologist.

Sexuality should receive special attention in young laryngectomees. These individuals generally have higher expectations of their sexual functioning, and often experience more negative impact of the laryngectomy on their sexual relationships than older laryngectomees. Specific attention should also be paid to other vulnerable persons, which include female laryngectomees, those with a lower educational background and laryngectomees with co-morbidity. These people are more at risk for a negative impact of the laryngectomy on their spousal relationship.

Chapter 17:

Imaging for detection and follow up (MRI, PET, and CT scans, X rays, and ultrasound)

Imaging techniques include Magnetic Resonance Imaging (MRI), Positron Emission Tomography (PET) scan, Computed Tomography (CT) scan, plain X rays, and ultrasound. All are non-invasive medical imaging procedures that enable the visualization of internal body structures. They are also used to detect cancer and follow up its progression and response to therapy.

Magnetic Resonance Imaging (MRI)

MRI can be used for cancer diagnosis, staging, and treatment planning. The main component of most MRI systems is a large tube-shaped or cylindrical magnet. Using non-ionizing radio frequency waves, powerful magnets, and a computer, this technology produces detailed, cross-sectional pictures of the inside of the body. In some cases, contrast dyes are used to illuminate certain structures in the body. These dyes may be injected directly into the bloodstream with a needle and syringe or they may be swallowed, depending on the area of the body being studied. With MRI, it is possible to distinguish between normal and diseased tissue and precisely pinpoint tumors within the body. It is also useful in detecting metastases. (**Picture 20**)

Additionally, the MRI provides greater contrast between the different soft tissues of the body than a CT scan. Thus, it is especially useful for imaging the brain, connective tissue, spine, muscles, and the inside of bones. To perform the scan the patient lies within a large device that creates magnetic field that aligns the magnetization of atomic nuclei in the body.

MRI tests are painless and there is no radiation involved. It takes much longer than a CT scan and is more expensive. Some patients report feelings of mild to severe anxiety and/or restlessness during the test. A mild sedative before the test can be administered to those who are claustrophobic or find it difficult to lie still for long periods of time. MRI machines produce loud banging, thumping, and humming sounds. Wearing earplugs can reduce the effect of noise.

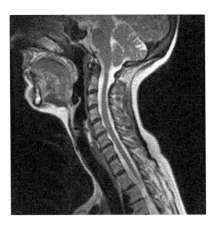

Picture 20: MRI of the head and neck

Computed Tomography (CT) Scan

CT scan is a medical imaging procedure that utilizes computer-processed series of X-rays to generate detailed tomographic images or 'cuts' of specific areas of the patient's body. These cross-sectional images are used for diagnostic and therapeutic purposes in many medical disciplines. (**Picture 21**) Digital geometry computerized processing is utilized to generate a three-dimensional image of the inside of a body site or organ from a large number of two-dimensional X-ray images taken around a single axis of rotation. Contrast dyes can be used to illuminate certain structures in the body. It is a quick test, but exposes the patient to radiation. Also dental work and movement during the procedure can distort the images.

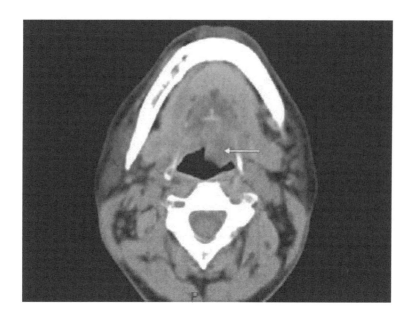

Picture 21: CT of the head and neck showing a cystic lesion

Positron Emission Tomography (PET)

PET scan is a nuclear medicine imaging test that creates a three-dimensional image or picture of the functional metabolic processes in the body. (**Picture 22**) It uses a radioactive substance called a "tracer" that is administered through a vein to look for disease in the body. The tracer travels through the blood and collects in organs and tissues with high metabolic activity. A single PET scan can accurately image the cellular function of the entire human body.

Since a PET scan detects increased metabolic activity of any cause, such as cancer, infection, or inflammation, it is not specific enough and therefore cannot differentiate between them. This can lead to equivocal interpretation of the results and may create uncertainty that can lead to further tests which may not be needed. In additional to the financial burden this can cause, it may generate anxiety and frustration.

It is also important to realize that these tests are not perfect and can miss a small tumor (less than one inch). A thorough physical examination should also accompany any scanning procedure.

PET and CT scans are often done in the same session and are performed by the same machine. While the PET scan demonstrates the biological function of the body, the CT scan provides information with respect to the location of any increased metabolic activity. By combining these two scanning technologies, a physician can more accurately diagnose and identify existing cancer.

The general recommendation is to perform fewer PET/CT scans the longer the elapsed time from the surgery that removed the cancer. Generally, PET/CT is performed every three to six months during the first year, then every six months during the second and then yearly throughout the fifth year. Some patients are followed yearly throughout life with PET/CT, and others undergo them if recurrence or a new malignancy is suspected. These recommendations, however, are not based on studies and are merely the opinion or consensus among the specialists. More scans are performed if there are concerns or suspicious findings. When scheduling a PET and/or CT scan any potential benefit gained by the information should be weighed against any potential deleterious effects of exposure to ionizing radiation and or X rays.

Sometimes physicians do not need a PET scan and only request a CT dedicated to the area in question. Such a CT is more precise compared to a combined PET/CT; the former can also include the injection of contrast material to assist in the diagnosis of the problem.

On occasion CT is not helpful, especially in those who had extensive dental work, including filings, crowns or implants that can interfere with the interpretation of the data. Not performing a CT spares the patient from receiving a substantial amount of radiation. Instead an MRI of the area can be done.

When viewing the scans, radiologists compare the new scan(s) with the old one's) to determine if there have been any changes. This can be useful in determining if there is new pathology.

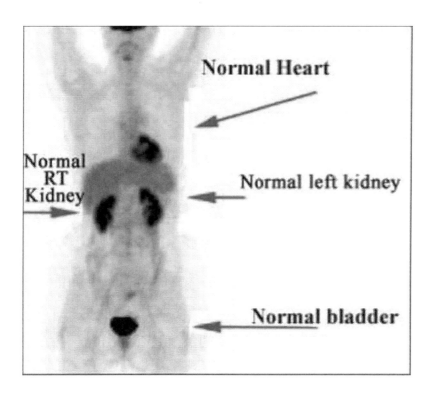

Picture 22: Normal PET scan

Plain X rays

X-radiation is an electromagnetic radiation produced by an X-ray tube. Plain X-rays radiography is an X-ray image generated by placing a body part in front of an X-ray detector and illuminating it with a short X-ray exposure. It is an inexpensive and easy method to evaluate the size of the heart and detect lung pathology including cancer spread.

Ultrasound

An ultrasound machine generates images that enables the examination of various body parts. The machine produces high-frequency sound waves through a hand held probe, which reflect off body structures. The handheld probe (called a transducer) is moved over the area being examined. A computer receives these reflected waves and creates a picture. There is no ionizing radiation exposure with this test. An ultrasound is a method that enables viewing vessels, structures and lymph nodes all over the body, including the neck and thyroid gland. It can also be used to obtain a biopsy of a lymph node or nodule.

Chapter 18:

Urgent care, CPR and care of laryngectomees during anesthesia

Rescue breathing for laryngectomees and other neck breathers

Laryngectomees and other neck breathers are at great risk of receiving inadequate acute care when they experience breathing difficulties or when they need cardiopulmonary resuscitation (CPR). Emergency departments (EDs) and emergency medical response services (EMS) personnel often do not recognize a patient who is a neck breather, do not know how to administer oxygen in the proper way, and may erroneously give mouth-to-mouth ventilation when mouth-to-stoma ventilation is indicated. This can lead to devastating consequences, depriving sick people from the oxygen needed to survive.

Many medical personnel are not familiar with the care of laryngectomees because a laryngectomy is a relatively rare procedure. Currently laryngeal cancers are detected and treated early. A total laryngectomy is generally indicated only for large tumors or for tumors that recur after previous treatment. There are currently only about 60 000 individuals who have undergone this procedure in the United States. As a result, acute care health providers have less contact than ever with laryngectomees.

This section outlines the special needs of laryngectomees and other neck breathers, explains the anatomical changes after laryngectomy, describes how laryngectomees speak and how to recognize them, outlines how to distinguish between total and partial neck breathers, and describes the procedures and equipment used in rescue breathing for total and partial neck breathers.

Causes of sudden respiratory distress in laryngectomees. The most common indication for a laryngectomy is cancer of the head and neck. Many laryngectomees also suffer from other medical problems resulting from their malignancy and its treatment which often includes radiation, surgery and chemotherapy. Laryngectomees also have difficulties in speaking and must therefore use various methods to communicate.

The most common cause of sudden breathing difficulty in laryngectomees is airway blockage due to aspiration foreign body or a mucus plug. laryngectomees may also suffer from other medical conditions including heart, lung and vascular problems.

The anatomy of after total laryngectomy. The anatomy of laryngectomees is different from the anatomy of those who have not undergone this procedure. **(Figure 1)** After a total laryngectomy, the patient breathes through a stoma (an opening in the neck for the trachea). There is no longer a connection between the trachea and the mouth and nose. Laryngectomees may be difficult to recognize because many cover their stomas with foam covers, ascots, or other garments. Many also apply a Heat and Moisture Exchanger (HME) or a Hands Free device over their stoma.

Differentiation between partial neck breathers and total neck breathers. It is important for medical personnel to differentiate partial neck breathers from total neck breathers (including laryngectomees) because the management of each group is different. The trachea is not connected to the upper airways in total neck breathers and all breathing is done through the tracheostomy site. In contrast, among partial neck breathers, although a tracheostomy site is present, there is still a connection between the trachea and the upper airways. Although partial neck breathers breathe mainly through their stoma, they are also able to breathe through their mouth and nose. The extent of breathing through the upper airways in these individuals varies.

Many partial neck breathers breathe through a tracheostomy tube, which may be protruding from the stoma and is often strapped to the neck. Failure to recognize a partial neck breather may lead to inappropriate treatment.

Preparation for rescue breathing. The steps to rescue a neck breather are:

1. Determine the patient's unresponsiveness
2. Activate the emergency medical services
3. Position the person by raising their shoulders
4. Expose the neck and remove anything covering the stoma such as filter or cloth that may prevent access to the airway
5. Secure the airway in the stoma and remove anything blocking the airway such as the filter or HME
6. Clear any mucus from the stoma.

It is not necessary to remove the stoma's housing unless it blocks the airway. Laryngectomy tubes or stoma buttons may be carefully removed. The voice prosthesis should not be removed, unless it is blocking the airway, since it generally does not interfere with breathing or suctioning. If the prosthesis is dislodged it should be removed and replaced with a catheter to prevent aspiration and fistula closure. If present, the tracheal tube may need to be suctioned after insertion of 2-5 cc of sterile saline or be entirely removed (both outer and inner parts) to clear any mucus plugs. The stoma should be wiped and suctioned. The next step is to listen for breathing sounds over the stoma. If the tracheostomy tube is blocked the chest may fail to rise.

If a tracheostomy tube is used for resuscitation it should be shorter than the regular one so that it can fit the length of the trachea. Care should be used in inserting the tube so that it does not dislodge the voice prosthesis. This may require the use of a tube with a smaller diameter.

If the patient is breathing normally he/she should be treated like any unconscious patient. If prolonged administration of oxygen is require, it should be humidified.

It may be difficult to detect a carotid artery pulse in the neck of some laryngectomees because of post radiation fibrosis. Some patients may not have a radial artery pulse in one of their arms if tissue from that arm was used for a free flap to reconstruct the upper airway.

Ventilation of total neck breathers. CPR for neck breathers is generally similar to CPR performed on normal individuals with one major exception. Neck breathers are administered ventilation and oxygen through their stoma. This can be done by a mouth-to-stoma ventilation or by using an oxygen mask (infant/toddler mask or an adult mask turned 90^0). (**Figure 7, Pictures 23 & 24**) It is useless to try to perform mouth-to-mouth ventilation.

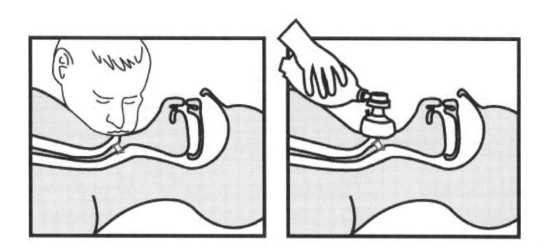

Figure 7: Ventilating a total neck breather

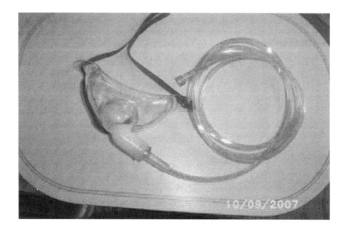

Picture 23: Oxygen mask

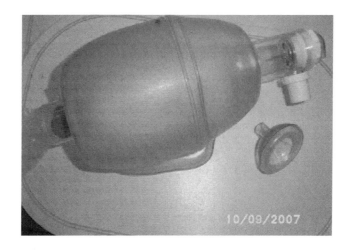

Picture 24: Infant bag valve mask used in rescue breathing

Ventilation of partial neck breathers. Although partial neck breathers inhale and exhale mainly through their stomas, they still have a connection between their lungs and their noses and mouths. (**Figure 8**) Therefore, air can escape from their mouths and/or noses, thus reducing the efficacy of ventilation. Even though partial neck breathers should receive ventilation through their stomas, their mouths should be kept closed and their noses sealed to prevent air from escaping. This can be done by holding the patient's mouth and nose tightly closed.

Partial Neck Breather
(Ventilate through stoma and occlude nose and mouth)

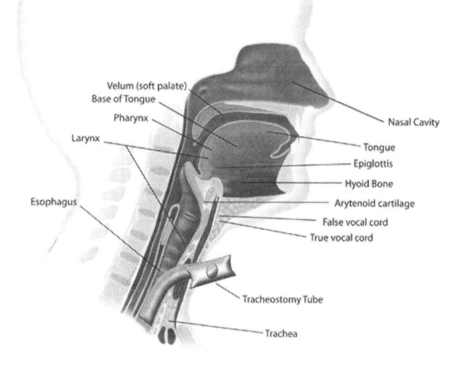

Figure 8: Anatomy of partial neck breather

Communication during respiratory distress

Laryngectomees may have difficulties in communication during respiratory distress and if possible they should be allowed to do so by writing or through flash cards. Laryngectomees and other neck breathers can assist in preventing life threatening mishaps by carrying an emergency card, displaying an emergency card in their car, and/or wearing a bracelet or a neck chain that identifies them as a neck breather. It is also important for them to carry a list of their medical conditions, the medication they take, the names of their doctors and contact information (see below). Laryngectomees should also communicate their unique needs ahead of time by calling the 911 services, the police department and the EMS in their community. They or their doctors should contact the EDs in their areas so that their personnel would be able to recognize neck breathers and deliver proper assistance to them.

Summary: Emergency department and EMS personnel should be vigilant in recognizing those who do not breathe through the mouth and nose. The knowledge of health care providers in communities may vary. Many health care providers are not familiar with the care of neck breathers, although this is taught at CPR courses. Proper administration of oxygen and ventilation through the stoma and specific details of CPR to neck breathers should be practiced periodically. The medical and EMS community should maintain their knowledge about the proper treatment of neck breathers so that effective care of these individuals is provided in urgent circumstances.

Respiratory problems unique to neck breathers include mucus plugs and foreign body aspiration. Although partial neck breathers inhale and exhale mainly through their stomas they still have a connection between their lungs, their noses, and their mouths. In contrast, there is no such connection in total neck breathers. Both partial and total neck breathers should be ventilated through their tracheostomy sites. However, the mouth needs to be closed and the nose sealed in partial neck breathers to prevent escape of air. An infant or toddler bag valve mask should be used in ventilating through the stoma.

Ensuring adequate urgent care for neck breathers including laryngectomees

Neck breathers are at a high risk of receiving inadequate therapy when seeking urgent medical care because of shortness of breath. It is common that medical personal mistakenly administer oxygen to the neck breather through their nose and not through their tracheotomy site.

Neck breathers can prevent a mishap by:

1. Wearing a bracelet that identifies them as neck breathers. (**Pictures 25 & 26**)
2. Carrying a list describing their medical conditions, their medication, the names of their doctors and their contact information.(**Picture 27**)
3. Have one's medical information and contacts in a health application on their android or IPhone.
4. Placing a sticker on the inside of their car windows identifying them as neck breathers. The card contains information about caring for them in an emergency.
5. Using an electrolarynx can be helpful and allow communication even in an emergency. Those who use a TEP for speech may not be able to speak because their HME may need to be removed.
6. Placing a note on their front door identifying themselves as a neck breather.
7. Informing the local 911 emergency services, EMSs and police department that they are neck breathers and may not be able to speak during an emergency.
8. Ensuring that the medical personnel of their local emergency rooms can recognize and treat neck breathers.

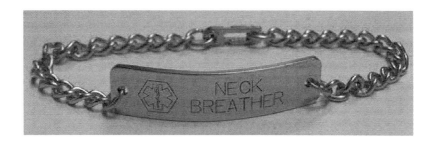

Picture 25: bracelet that identifies a neck breathers

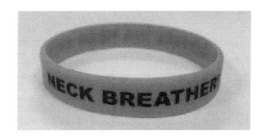

Picture 26: bracelet that identifies a neck breathers

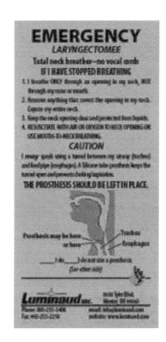

Picture 27: A card describing the medical conditions, medication, the names of one's medical providers and their contact information

It is up to laryngectomees to be vigilant and increase the awareness of the medical personnel and EMSs in their area. This can be an ongoing task, since knowledge by health providers may vary and change over time.

A video presentation of rescue breathing can be watched on YouTube at https://goo.gl/Unstch

Neck breathers should share these presentations with their emergency care givers (Closest ED and EMS).

Undergoing a procedure or surgery as a laryngectomee

Undergoing a procedure, (e.g., colonoscopy) by sedation or surgery by either local or general anesthesia is challenging for laryngectomees.

Unfortunately, most medical personnel who care for laryngectomees before, during, and after surgery are not familiar with their unique anatomy, how they speak, and how to manage their airways during and after the procedure or operation. These include nurses, medical technicians, surgeons and even anesthetists.

It is therefore advisable that laryngectomees explain their unique needs and anatomy beforehand the surgery to those who will be treating them. Using explanatory illustrations or pictures is helpful. Those with voice prostheses should allow their anesthetist to view their stoma in order to understand its function and be warned not to remove it. It is helpful to provide the anesthetist a video that illustrates how to ventilate neck breather (send a request to customersupport.us@atosmedical.com), or provide them with the link to it on YouTube at: https://goo.gl/Unstch

Medical personnel should understand that an individual with a total laryngectomy has no connection between the oropharynx and the trachea and therefore ventilation and airway suctioning should be done through the stoma and not through the nose or mouth.

Undergoing a procedure with sedation or surgery under local anesthesia is challenging for a laryngectomee because speaking with an electrolarynx or voice prosthesis is generally not possible. This is because the stoma is covered by an oxygen mask and the patient's hands are typically bound. However, individuals who use esophageal speech can communicate throughout the procedure or surgery done under local anesthesia.

It is important to discuss one's special requirements with the medical team prior to surgery. This may require repeating it several times, first to surgeons, than to the anesthetist in the pre surgical evaluation, and lastly on the day of surgery to the anesthesia team that is actually going to be in the operating room. If possible, one could coordinate with the anesthetist prior to the surgery how to notify him/her of pain, or the need to be suctioned. Hand signals, head nodding, lip reading or sounds produced by rudimentary esophageal speech can be helpful.

Using these suggestions may help laryngectomees get adequate care whenever they undergo a medical procedures or surgery done under local anesthesia.

Cardio-Pulmonary Resuscitation (CPR) new guidelines

The new American Heart association CPR 2012 guidelines require only cardiac compressions; mouth to mouth breathing is no longer necessary. The main purpose of the new guidelines is to encourage more people to deliver CPR. Many individuals avoid mouth to mouth resuscitation because they feel inhibited by breathing into someone's mouth or nose. The impetus for the new guidelines is that it is better to use the chest compressions method only rather than doing nothing.

An official video that demonstrates the Hands-Only CPR is available at:
https://www.youtube.com/watch?v=zSgmledxFe8

Because laryngectomees cannot administer mouth to mouth breathing the old CPR guidelines excluded them from providing the respiratory part of CPR. Since the new guidelines do not require mouth to mouth ventilation laryngectomees can also deliver CPR. However, when possible the old CPR method using both airway ventilation and cardiac compressions should be utilized. This is because the "chest compressions only" method cannot sustain someone for a long period of time since there is no aeration of the lungs.

Laryngectomees who require CPR may also need respiratory ventilation. One of the common causes of breathing problems in laryngectomees is airway obstruction due to a mucus plug or foreign body. Removing these may be essential. Mouth to stoma resuscitation is important and relatively easier to deliver than mouth to mouth breathing.

Laryngectomees who breathe through a Heat and Moisture Exchanger (HME) and perform CPR on a person in need of resuscitation may need to temporarily take their HME off. This allows laryngectomees to inhale more air when they deliver up to one hundred heart compressions per minute.

Chapter 19:

Travelling and driving as a laryngectomee

Traveling and driving as a laryngectomee can be challenging. The trip may expose the traveler to unfamiliar places away from their routine and comfortable settings. Laryngectomees may need to care for their airways at unfamiliar locations. Traveling usually requires planning ahead so that essential supplies are available during the trip. It is important to continue to care for one's airways and other medical issues while travelling.

Driving a car as a laryngectomee

Driving a car can be challenging for a laryngectomee. Speaking may be difficult while driving because of the noise produced by the car and the traffic.

Holding the steering wheel with two hands is essential for safe driving. However, speaking using an electrolarynnx or voice prosthesis (with a non-hands free HME) requires the use of one's hand. This leaves the driver with only a single hand to steer and operate their car. Using hands free Heat and Moisture Exchanger (HME) frees both hands to continue and operate the car.

Another potential problem is the need to cough or sneeze while driving. The air inhaled when driving busy roads and highways is often polluted and may cause respiratory irritation and coughing. The sputum produced by coughing or sneezing can block the HME cassette and prevent breathing. Laryngectomees need to quickly remove the blocked HME to allow breathing. This requires using their hand(s) and creates a dangerous situation.

Safer driving can be enhanced by:

- Pulling over to the curb when experiencing coughing or sneezing, or when needing to speak (when using an electrolarynx or non-hands free HME)
- Do not use your cell phone (even a hands free one) while driving
- Stopping frequently to cough out one's sputum
- Using Hands Free HME while driving
- Avoiding direct exposure to outside air while driving by using the car's ventilation
- Making sure that the car's safety belts do no impede breathing by covering your stoma
- Roll up the car windows, and use the air condition to reduce exposure to dust and irritants

Laryngectomees who use an electrolarynx need to be careful if they are stopped by a policeman. The electrolarynx may be mistaken for a weapon by the policeman. It is advisable not to get hold of it until one can explain to the policeman that they need the electrolarynx to speak. This can be done by handing over a written explanation.

Risk associated with deployment of inflatable airbag

Inflatable airbag can prevent serious injury and can save lives. The airbag provides the occupants a soft cushioning and restraint during a crash and prevents any impact injury with the interior of the vehicle. Unfortunately, in neck breathers including laryngectomees, the deployment of inflatable airbag may block air access to the stoma. Consideration should be given to measures that may preventing this occurrence.

These measures include having the laryngectomee sit in a rear seat, and measures that can provide an adequate distance between the driver and the steering wheel (e.g., moving the seat rearward, inclining the seat back, adjusting a telescoping steering wheel toward the dashboard). Information about these measures can be obtained from the National Mobility Dealers Association at 1-800-833-0427.

Disconnecting the airbag all together should be discouraged as their benefit outweighs the potential risk. However, neck breathers should consult their physician about this option.

Caring for the airways while flying on a commercial airline

Taking a flight (especially a long one) on a commercial airline presents several challenges.

Several factors can lead to deep vein thrombosis or DVT. These include insufficient hydration (due to low moisture in the cabin air at high altitude), lower oxygen pressure inside the plane, and the passenger's immobility. These factors, when combined, can cause a blood clot in the legs that, when dislodged, can circulate through the blood stream and reach the lungs where it can cause pulmonary embolism. This is a serious complication and a medical emergency.

 In addition, low air humidity can dry out the trachea and lead to mucus plugs. Airline attendants are typically unfamiliar with the means of providing air to a laryngectomee (i.e., directing air to the stoma and not the nose).

These steps can be taken to prevent potential problems:

- Drinking at least 8 ounces of water for every two hours on a plane, including ground time
- Avoiding alcohol and caffeine drinks, as they are dehydrating
- Wearing loose-fitting clothes
- Avoiding crossing one's legs while seating, as this can reduce blood flow in the legs
- Wearing compression socks
- If in a higher risk category, asking one's doctor whether to take aspirin before flying to inhibit blood clotting
- Performing legs exercises and standing up or walking, whenever possible during the flight
- Booking a seat in an exit row, bulkhead, or aisle seat that allows greater leg room

- Informing the flight attendants that one is a laryngectomee
- Placing medical supplies, including stoma care equipment and an electrolarynx (if used) in an accessible place in the carry-on luggage (It is allowed to bring durable medical equipment and supplies on board, even as an extra carry-on bag)
- Communicating with flight attendants through writing if the noise during the flight make it difficult to speak
- Inserting saline into your stoma periodically during the flight to keep the trachea moist
- Covering the stoma with a Heat and Moisture Exchanger (HME) or a moist cloth to provide humidity

These measures make airline travel easier and safer for laryngectomees and other neck breathers.

Supplies to carrying when travelling

When travelling it is useful to carry all one's airways management supplies and medication in a dedicated bag. The bag should not be checked in and access to it should be easy.

Suggested items to be included in the bag include:

- A summary of one's medication taken on a regular basis, one's medical diagnoses and allergies, the names and contact information of one's medical providers, a referral to a speech and language pathologist (SLP), and prescriptions for one's medication
- Proof of medical and dental insurance
- A supply of the medications taken
- Paper tissues
- Tweezers, mirror, flash light (with extra batteries)
- Blood pressure monitor (for those who are hypertensive)

- Saline bullets
- Supplies for placing HME housing (alcohol, Remove, Skin Tag, glue)
- Several HMEs and HME housings
- Carrying an electrolarynx (with extra batteries) even by those using a voice prosthesis may be helpful in case one is unable to speak
- A voice amplifier (if needed, with extra batteries or a battery charger)

Individuals who use a voice prosthesis should also bring these items:

- An extra hands free HME and an extra voice prosthesis
- A brush and flushing bulb to clean one's voice prosthesis
- A red Foley catheter (to place in the voice prosthesis' puncture in case the voice prosthesis is dislodged)

The quantity of supply items depends on the length of the trip.

It can be useful to obtain contact information for SLP(s) and physicians at the area of travel.

Preparing a kit with essential information and material when going to the hospital

Laryngectomees may need to receive emergency and non-emergency medical care at a hospital or other medical facility. Because of their difficulty in communicating with medical personnel and providing information, especially when in distress it is helpful to prepare a folder with this information. Additionally it is useful to carry a kit containing items and supplies needed to maintain their ability to communicate and care for their stoma. The kit should be kept in a place that is easily accessible in an emergency.

The kit should contain the following:

- An updated and current summary of the medical and surgical history, allergies and diagnoses
- An updated list of the medications taken and the results of all procedures, radiological examinations, scans and laboratory tests. These may be placed on a disc or USB flash drive
- Contact information and proof of medical insurance
- Information (phone, email, address) of the laryngectomee's physician(s), speech and language pathologist, family members and friend(s)
- A figure or drawing of a side view of the neck that explains the anatomy of the laryngectomee's upper airways and if relevant where the voice prosthesis is located
- A paper pad and pen
- An electrolarynx with extra batteries (even for those using a voice prosthesis)
- A box of paper tissues
- A supply of saline bullets, HME filters, HME housing, and supplies needed to apply and remove them (e.g., alcohol, Remove, Skin Tag, glue) and to clean the voice prosthesis (brush, flushing bulb)
- Tweezers, mirror, flash light (with extra batteries)

Having these items available when seeking emergency or regular care can be critically important.

ADDENDUM

Useful resources:

- American cancer society information on head and neck cancer at: http://www.cancer.gov/cancertopics/types/head-and-neck/
- United Kingdom cancer support site on head and neck cancer at: http://www.macmillan.org.uk/Cancerinformation/Cancertypes/Larynx/Laryngealcancer.aspx#.UJGZu8V9lxg
- International Association of Laryngectomees at: http://www.theial.com/ial/
- Oral Cancer Foundation at: http://oralcancerfoundation.org/
- Mouth Cancer Foundation at: http://www.mouthcancerfoundation.org/
- Support for People with Oral and Head and Neck Cancer at: http://www.spohnc.org/
- A site that contains useful links for laryngectomees and other head and neck cancer patients at: http://www.bestcancersites.com/laryngeal/
- My Voice-Itzhak Brook MD information Website at: http://dribrook.blogspot.com/
- Head and Neck Cancer Alliance at: http://www.headandneck.org/
- Head and Neck Cancer Alliance Support Community at: http://www.inspire.com/groups/head-and-neck-cancer-alliance/
- WebWhispers at: http://www.webwhispers.org/

Laryngectomees groups in Facebook:

- Laryngectomy Support
- Strictly speaking a laryngectomy
- Survivors of head and neck cancer

- Throat and oral cancer survivors
- Head and neck cancer survivors
- Support for People with Oral and Head and Neck Cancer (SPOHNC)
- Webwhispers

List of the major medical suppliers for laryngectomees:

- Atos Medical: http://www.atosmedical.us/
- Bruce Medical Supplies: http://www.brucemedical.com/
- Fahl Medizintechnik: http://www.fahl-medizintechnik.de/
- Griffin Laboratories: http://www.griffinlab.com/
- InHealth Technologies: http://store.inhealth.com/
- Lauder The Electrolarynx Company: http://www.electrolarynx.com/
- Luminaud Inc.: http://www.luminaud.com/
- Romet Electronic larynx: http://www.romet.us/
- Ultravoice: http://www.ultravoice.com/

ABOUT THE AUTHOR

Dr. Itzhak Brook is a physician who specializes in pediatrics and infectious diseases. He is a Professor of Pediatrics at Georgetown University Washington D.C. and his areas of expertise are anaerobic and head and neck infections including sinusitis. He has done extensive research on respiratory tract infections and infections following exposure to ionizing radiation. Dr Brook served in the US Navy for 27 years. He is the author of six medical textbooks, 150 medical book chapters and over 750 scientific publications. He is an editor of three and associate editor of four medical journals. Dr. Brook is the author of "My Voice-a Physician's Personal Experience with Throat Cancer" and "In the Sands of Sinai-a Physician's Account of the Yom-Kippur War". He is a board member of the Head and Neck Cancer Alliance. Dr. Brook is the recipient of the 2012 J. Conley Medical Ethics Lectureship Award by the American Academy of Otolaryngology-Head and Neck Surgery. Dr. Brook was diagnosed with throat cancer in 2006.

IV Pole Not Req - have bag above head
gravity Drip

oram   Page 22 -

Cases   if tube is out of place (stitch in nose)
        Days   go to ER
24 = 4+2 feedings

~~F~~   be careful put on, take of cloths

2 cases formula
                        Reclining + upright is ok - for his position

10 sets

8'⁰ Syringes   Nutrition Program

                       Room Temp   No refrigeration

                       2 weeks from date of surgery - until follow up appt

                       No H₂O till then.

                              flush tube w H₂O before + after

                       get rid of air in tube
                       Roll the clamp to get formula to

               Trash the feeding set end of day

               Syringes - wash warm H₂O + soap
                          can re use

Made in the USA
Middletown, DE
11 January 2021